This Can't Happen to Me!

This Can't Happen to Me!

Tackling Type 2 diabetes

Tim Bowden

ALLEN&UNWIN

First published in 2004 by Allen & Unwin

Allen & Unwin
83 Alexander Street
Crows Nest NSW 2065
Australia
Phone: (61 2) 8425 0100
Fax: (61 2) 9906 2218
Email: info@allenandunwin.com
Web: www.allenandunwin.com

National Library of Australia
Cataloguing-in-Publication entry:

Bowden, Tim, 1937- .
This can't happen to me! : tackling type 2 diabetes.

ISBN 1 74114 318 7.

1. Bowden, Tim, 1937- . 2. Diabetes - Biography. 3. Non-insulin-dependent diabetes. 4. Diabetes - Australia. I. Title.

362.1964620092

Set in 12/16 pt Adobe Garamond Pro by Bookhouse, Sydney

10 9 8 7 6 5 4 3 2 1

Foreword

It's an irony that I sit and write this on the 100th anniversary of the Wright brothers taking flight in North Carolina. It launched a technology that profoundly changed our lives in what seems to be the blink of an eye. But air travel is just one of the changes to our lives since then. The world that Orville and Wilbur Wright were born into still had smallpox; TB (tuberculosis) was rife—in fact the organism which causes it had been discovered only a few years before they pushed off at Kitty Hawk; there was a plague epidemic (yes, the Black Death) spreading around the Pacific islands; and life expectancy was 47 years. Heart attacks were as rare as hen's teeth; children with Type 1 diabetes died because the use of insulin was still a couple of decades away; and while Type 2 diabetes did exist, it would have been pretty uncommon, and not often recognised as the cause of rotten feet, blindness and kidney failure.

People often ask me what there is to worry about these days when, despite the agonising headlines about obesity and Type 2 diabetes, we are living longer and longer. The first thing to say about this is that we shouldn't be complacent. A major event in recent history showed us that life expectancy can be thrown into reverse. When the Berlin Wall came down it wasn't just the concrete that tumbled: a social and political tidal wave swept across the former Soviet countries of Eastern Europe. From Berlin to Vladivostock, life expectancy rapidly fell to below the levels of some developing nations. There's no guarantee that things will always become better just because they have in the past.

The second factor is that the experts no longer call Type 2 diabetes 'adult onset', because children are now being diagnosed with it. No-one knows what impact this will have on our longevity.

Thirdly, it's high technology and expensive medicine that are keeping things in check when prevention can work. Lose the access to these and where are we?

Although Orville and Wilbur devoted themselves to easier, faster transportation, they still walked or cycled to the shops, their washing was done by hand and in general hard physical work was more common than it is now. Our obesity and diabetes epidemics are epidemics of plenty (of calorie-dense foods) on the one hand and of scarcity (of adequate exercise) on the other. We're talking about an epidemic of muscle deficiency. Apart from the brain, muscle is just about the most metabolically active tissue in the body. It's better to be fat with muscle than fat and floppy.

Now I'd never call Tim fat and floppy—at least never to his face—and certainly not after he's invented his new sleek self in response to the diagnosis that made him write about his experiences for my radio program and this book. But Tim did partake in a lot of what the modern world had to offer. He was one of the first people I met after joining the ABC and he freely gave advice to this new boy about everything from cut-editing magnetic tape and filling out ABC expense sheets (I've since passed that on to many), to where to have a decent lunch or a drink after work. Tim could extract the finer things in life wherever he went and could suck every last nutrient from a Thai meal (his and others'), but one place he never went was the gym.

How things have changed.

This book will be immensely valuable to people with Type 2 diabetes, young and silver-haired. There's nothing like sharing a person's journey to assist your own. As always Tim is showing the road, if somewhat more ascetically than in the past.

Dr Norman Swan
Host, *The Health Report,* ABC Radio National
17 December 2003

Contents

Acknowledgements

If Dr Norman Swan had not asked me to write a series of talks for ABC Radio National's *Health Report* in March 2003, following my unexpected—isn't that always the way?—diagnosis with Type 2 diabetes, this book is unlikely to have been written. Annette Barlow, publisher at Allen & Unwin, happened to hear some of them and asked me to consider writing a book drawing on my own experiences and those of other Type 2s to raise awareness of this often hidden disease. So thank you Norman and Annette for entrenching me on a faster learning curve on diabetes than I might otherwise have embarked on.

This book has been enhanced by the frank way my fellow Type 2s have shared their own stories and experiences with this unforgiving, incurable condition. I thank all contributors who are named in the narrative.

I have had unstinting help and assistance from Diabetes Australia–NSW, and have plundered their expertise mercilessly. Dr Lilian Jackson, DA's Health and Education Division manager, not only agreed to be interviewed but nobly accepted the time-consuming task of checking the manuscript for accuracy in both medical and general aspects of diabetes. Bill Edmunds, DA's NSW Manager of Corporate Relations and Communications, was a powerhouse of ideas, historical sources and the intricate politics of diabetes. Thanks also to Alan Barclay, a dietitian at Diabetes Australia–NSW, who steered me through the thorny dietary thickets of the glycaemic index and 'good' and 'bad' cholesterol. Truly we are what we eat. Diabetes Australia–NSW also allowed me to reproduce some of their excellent published information, which is much appreciated.

Professor Lesley Campbell, the Director of the Diabetes Centre at St Vincent's Hospital in Sydney and a world renowned researcher into diabetes, cheerfully disrupted her punishing schedule to talk to me about many aspects of Type 2, ranging from sex to the possibilities of a future cure for this stubborn and intractable disease. I am indebted to Dr Kerry Bowen, an endocrinologist at Royal Newcastle Hospital, for a succinct and user-friendly rundown on the modern drugs used to treat Type 2 diabetes. I particularly appreciated the help and sage advice from my fellow scribe, Harry Robinson, now retired in Canberra, who has late onset diabetes for two decades and was able to assuage many of my fears shortly after I was diagnosed.

Back at the ranch at Allen & Unwin, Jemma Birrell speedily and accurately typed up transcripts of my recorded interviews. Managing Editor Rebecca Kaiser (for whom there is never a problem that cannot be overcome) was encouraging and unstinting with her time and advice as always. I also thank Simon Paterson at Bookhouse for designing such a distinctive and elegant text and Nada Backovic for a wonderful cover.

My local GP, Ron, has had to put up with me as an

interviewer as well as a patient, and did so with his usual good cheer. Dr Ian Adair, CEO of the Alliance of NSW Divisions, weighed in with little notice on behalf of the GPs who are on the frontline of the diagnosis and treatment of diabetes, and copped criticism—as well as praise—from some of the Type 2s I interviewed.

I should also not forget to thank diabetes educator, David Mapletoft, who contacted me after hearing my ABC *Health Report* broadcasts, to suggest I consider sharing my experiences in other media.

Special thanks are due to my wife Ros who was her usual supportive self during my (mercifully brief) despair and hypochondria phase, and has also joined me on a diabetes friendly diet, creating wondrously interesting and nutritious dishes. And if I am tempted to stray from the true and virtuous path, diabetes nurse educator Ivy Semple and dietitian John Jones will help Ros keep me on the straight and narrow through their excellent work at the Forster Community Health Centre, on the mid north coast of NSW.

Acknowledgements are the hardest part of a book to write, because there are always horrific omissions that you only discover after publication. To anyone I've missed, I'm sorry and thank you.

CHAPTER ONE

But I'm bulletproof . . .

It seemed a good idea at the time. I had turned 65 and I thought I should have a medical once-over, including a fasting blood test to screen the function of every organ, from my prostate to my long-suffering liver. Let's face it, most journalists are not unfond of a drink and traditionally give their livers a bit of a work-over. As it turned out, mine was a bit inflamed—poor thing—and I felt a bit disappointed with it. It had let me down at a crucial moment. But it was the performance of my pancreas that had my normally phlegmatic GP unusually animated.

'Your blood glucose reading is very high,' he said.

'Never mind,' I said smugly. 'I'll be a good boy, lose some weight, do some more exercise and we'll try it again in a few months.'

This response actually had Ron leaping out of his chair. 'No we won't', he said grimly. 'With a reading of 9.8 [mmol/L][1] you've almost certainly got diabetes. What we'll do right now is order up a glucose tolerance test that will tell me definitively whether you have diabetes or not!'

A diabetic, me?

I was confident I could prove him wrong. No Bowden had ever had diabetes, nor, as far as I could remember, had there been diabetes in my mother's family. I remember my wife Ros saying that her grandfather had diabetes, and used to order in a case of 'diabetic whisky' fairly regularly for therapeutic reasons. Well I wasn't related to him, but it sounded like a good idea. I'd never heard of diabetic whisky. But that was because, as I was to find out later, no such joy juice existed.

I wasn't even sure what having diabetes meant as far as my health was concerned, except that the news wasn't likely to be good. But I didn't see any point in asking questions about it unless I needed to. Clearly I'd had the fasting blood test at an unfortunate time; it must have been after that indulgent dinner party. I looked forward to disabusing Ron of his absurd belief that I might have diabetes.

The glucose tolerance test involved a lot of blood taking. Hungry and irritable with no breakfast to sustain me, I drove to my nearest pathology clinic. I took a trailer load of garden clippings to take to the tip so as not to waste the trip to town—these days I live in what Prime Minister John Howard refers to as, 'reejunal and rooral Austraya', on the mid north coast of New South Wales—but to my surprise the clinic wouldn't let

---

1 millimoles per litre

me out of their sight. After the first blooding I was given a bottle of sweet, fizzy stuff to drink. I was told I had 15 minutes to get it inside me, but I gurgled it down in 15 seconds.

'Why can't I go off to the tip with my trailer and come back in three-quarters of an hour?'

'Because any physical activity can influence your test result.'

So I had to while away the next two hours with two more blood samples by reading the book I'd mercifully brought with me.

That night I went out, defiantly, to partake in an eight-course Chinese banquet, complete with Peking duck and lashings of wine. I told my friend Malcolm, a large food- and wine-loving feller, of the Sword of Diabetes hanging over me because of the high blood sugar reading.

'Oh, that happened to me', he said. (Malcolm was an engineer by trade, and so is blessed with total certainty about everything.) 'I realised my high reading was caused by drinking sweet apple juice before breakfast. I swapped it for tomato juice and everything was fine.'

Ron suggested I bring Ros in when I came back to see him two days later—he must have been fairly sure he had bad news to deliver. Sitting in front of his GP's desk I eyeballed him sternly.

'Now before you tell me anything, I want you to know that I've found out what the problem is and I've fixed it.' I told him Malcolm's apple and tomato juice story, but he was unimpressed.

'Bullshit', he said. 'It's not the apple juice or any other fruit juice, it's how your body copes with sugar, glucose, all the time, not just at breakfast. And I have to tell you that the glucose tolerance test you've just had is a conclusive test on whether you have diabetes or not. Not to put too fine a point on it, your results are lousy.'

He leaned forward across his desk. 'Listen to me, Tim, and watch my lips. You . . . have . . . Type 2 diabetes. You . . . are . . . a . . . diabetic.

'That's the bad news. The good news is that this is not a death sentence, it is in fact a life sentence. Type 2 diabetes can often be controlled by diet and exercise, at least initially. You need to start eating low-fat, low-sugar food, do more exercise and lose about ten kilos. I don't think you will have to take any drugs specifically for diabetes at this stage, but I don't know that for sure yet, until we test you again in three months. However, you will probably have to go on some medication for diabetes eventually.'

He went on, 'Type 2 diabetes occurs when the insulin your body produces is less efficient at controlling blood glucose levels. This is called "insulin resistance". Associated with insulin resistance is high blood pressure and elevated cholesterol levels, which could lead to heart disease or strokes. Your kidneys might also be affected. You will need to get your eyes tested once a year, and your feet checked over by a podiatrist regularly, as they also suffer from the effects of your condition. I'm going to increase your anti-cholesterol medication and put you on tablets to bring your blood pressure down.'

Then, the bombshell:

'You can have no more than three "standard" alcoholic drinks a day. Some say only two, but I sense that you might need three, although it would be better if you gave it up completely. You should have at least two alcohol-free days a week.'

'Alcohol-free days?' I yelped. 'I haven't had one of those since I left school!'

'You'll get used to it. And I want you to prick your fingers twice a day and use a blood-sugar testing machine you can get from the chemist and keep a record of the results. And, get used to the fact that you have diabetes. You will always have diabetes. What you have to do is manage it sensibly.'

My thoughts were straying to the concept of a standard drink. I couldn't ever remember having one. After a day like this four decent-sized ones sounded a bit light on. 'But I haven't had any symptoms.'

'That's right. People can have it for years and not know. You are one of the lucky ones, being diagnosed early.'

I didn't feel lucky. 'What happens if I don't do anything about it?'

'Well it's a long list, Tim. Where do you want me to start? Cardiovascular disease leading to a heart attack or strokes. You'll almost certainly have problems with your eyesight. I mentioned damage to your kidneys before, and we might as well throw your liver in for good measure. Other things you can look forward to, if you ignore your diabetes, are loss of sensation and pain in your feet—and with poor circulation caused by cardiovascular problems this can lead to amputations of toes, feet or even your lower legs. Shall I go on?'

I knew Ron was an up-front no-nonsense GP, which is one of the reasons I go to him. But I was looking for the good news. Still in shock, I suddenly realised I was due to leave on a voyage to the Antarctic Peninsula in five weeks' time. Could I still go?

Ron said he thought I probably would be able to travel, but it depended on how my blood sugars reacted to the new regime. 'I normally give people a bit of time to get used to the idea before starting them on a blood testing regime, but the sooner you get cracking on that the sooner I'll know whether you can go to Antarctica or not. So you can start tonight.'

He recommended a chemist who stocked the blood glucose testing meter I would need, wrote a scrip for the lancets and my first testing strips, advised me to join the National Diabetes Services Scheme managed by Diabetes Australia, and prepared to receive his next patient. 'Cheer up', he said as I mooched out. 'Remember what I said. It's not a death sentence—it's a life sentence.'

'Terrific', I thought.

Ros and I didn't go home but drove straight to our nearest town, Forster, 30 kilometres away, to the recommended pharmacy. I began to realise I was in diabetic heartland, the coastal retirement belt. The chemist even had a special person in charge of their diabetes section who took me under her wing.

'You're in luck today,' she said brightly. 'We've got a very good machine on special with 40 per cent off.'

I wondered dimly why everyone kept telling me I was lucky.

'You'll also need to sign up with the National Diabetes Services Scheme, which will allow you to get testing strips and other diabetic necessities at a discount. I've got the forms here, so let's do it now.'

Feeling as though this was happening to someone else, I filled in the form while Jeannie snapped a small electronic blood glucose testing machine out of its box, and uncapped a cylinder of testing strips. Whipping one out, she popped it into the end of the meter. It was a thin plastic strip about five centimetres long with a copper electrode on one end, and a little yellow indentation at the other with an absorbent pad to soak up my blood.

The kit had a pen-sized spring-loaded lancet, which Jeannie loaded by pushing down a button on the end—rather like a retractable biro. It also had a numbered cylinder on the business end, from 1 to 5, depending on how deep the needle needed to go. She showed me how to fire it into the side of a finger, near the nail where the blood supply was readily available, and not the finger tips which might get sore. With two pricks a day, I thought I was going to run out of fingers quite soon, but Jeannie explained you could return to a pricked digit within a day or so.

Without further ado I felt a slight sting on the side of my forefinger and the bubble of blood that obligingly appeared was soaked up by the little yellow pad on the test strip she'd inserted into the blood-testing meter. A zero danced around the screen. After about seven seconds, it produced a reading of 7.9—I didn't know whether that was good or bad. A bit on the high side actually, I discovered, but these were early days. Jeannie then produced a little diary and showed me where to record my blood sugar levels at various times of the day: before meals, and two hours after eating. Not before and after every meal, I was relieved to hear, but two tests each day, staggered, to give a wide coverage during the week.

I stumbled out into the early afternoon with my new machine, enough testing strips and pricking lancets to go on with, my marked-up diary and a fuddled brain. What I needed was a pie with sauce, a vanilla slice and a soft drink to wash it down, all forbidden from now on. For ever.

My sympathetic but practical spouse whipped up a lettuce salad with cottage cheese and three-bean mix. It was likely to be a windy afternoon. I washed that down with soda water and indulged in a slice of wholegrain bread with a thin slice of cheese and a smidgeon of honey, then munched mournfully on an apple.

Two hours after digesting this rabbit food, I had to prick myself to monitor my blood sugar to see how my body had absorbed what, by my standards, could hardly be called a decent lunch. I loaded up the pricker and fired into the side of my left index finger. I felt a sting, but no blood appeared. So I loaded and fired again, into my forefinger. A slight bubble of blood appeared, but not enough, as I quickly discovered, to fully saturate the test strip, thus giving a false reading. I wound up the penetration gauge to its maximum setting of 5 and, in some frustration, fired again at the side of my little finger. This time my pinky yielded up enough of the claret to satisfy the machine.

'Ha, ha', I thought positively, 'I'll change the needle', which must have been blunt by now. As I picked up the pricker and tried to remove the cap that Jeannie in the pharmacy had so deftly clicked into place, the whole thing disintegrated. As it did so, it fired its unsheathed dart right into the tip of my forefinger, unleashing a spurt of blood that sprayed, to my surprise, half a metre across the kitchen bench and all over the front of my blood test diary, an enduring stain and bloody reminder of my first ham-fisted attempts at self-testing. I seemed to be the Lady Macbeth of the BGL (blood glucose level) meter.[2]

I needed to know more about diabetes, and the information summarised in the Diabetes Australia pamphlet was a sobering read. There are 1.2 million people in Australia with diabetes, and half of them don't know they've got it! Diabetes is the world's

---

2 'Out, damned spot! . . . who would have thought the old man to have had so much blood in him?' *Macbeth*, Act V, Scene I (After the murder of King Duncan, Lady Macbeth sleep walks and tries to wash Duncan's blood from her hands.)

fastest-growing disease. In Australia alone, 214 people are diagnosed every day, and diabetes is the seventh highest contributing cause of death in Australia.

The vast majority, 90 per cent or so, have, like me, Type 2 diabetes, which can be controlled by diet, exercise and, in some cases, regular medication. People with Type 1 diabetes have to inject themselves with insulin around two to four times a day, and monitor their blood glucose levels extremely carefully, lest their levels drop so low they have a 'hypo' (see box). Or if they allow their blood sugar levels to get too high they can have an equally dangerous 'hyper' (see box). Those with Type 2 diabetes are only at risk of a hypo if they are on insulin or certain medications.

Hypoglycaemia—hypos

Hypos, or low blood glucose levels, can happen when blood glucose levels drop to below 4 mmol/L. The person then may begin to feel unwell, become pale, sweaty and shaky and present with abnormal behaviour. If left untreated this may progress to loss of consciousness and, in some cases, death.

Treatment should be immediate and a sweet drink or lolly, such as a glucose sweet or jelly beans, should be given, followed by a snack. No food should be given to an unconscious person—call for an ambulance.

Hypos can occur in people with Type 1 diabetes because they have taken too much insulin, not eaten enough or had too much physical activity.

Hypos can also occur in Type 2 diabetes for people on certain oral medications and insulin.

Hyperglycaemia—hypers

Hypers happen when blood glucose levels rise too high. This can occur when a person does not take enough diabetes medication, whether it is tablets or insulin. Stress and infections or other illness, as well as some medications, can also cause blood sugar levels to increase.

As the blood glucose level rises, symptoms will include passing lots of urine, a dry mouth, excessive thirst, blurred vision and tiredness. Some people do not feel all or even any of these hyper symptoms if blood sugar levels are not yet very high. However if a hyper is not treated, people with Type 1 diabetes may develop vomiting, nausea and abdominal pain, symptoms of ketoacidosis, which can be life threatening.

Ketoacidosis—where acidic by-products called ketones can build up in the blood, and some pass into the urine—are much more common with Type 1s but can occur, uncommonly, with Type 2s under certain circumstances. (Ketones can be detected by the use of urine testing strips.) If there is a severe lack of insulin, vomiting can result which increases dehydration.

This is a serious medical problem and must be treated urgently by referral to hospital and specialist services.

I read that Type 2 diabetics are, at least sometimes, but not always, spared the injection routine. But the complications of the disease are dire, particularly if untreated. It's the most common cause of blindness in people over 60 and the number one cause of kidney failure. Diabetics are two to four times more likely to develop heart disease than non-diabetics. In fact 65 to 80 per cent of us will die of coronary heart disease. And if that wasn't bad enough, we might be taken off by a stroke, and before that, have our feet amputated because of poor circulation and nerve damage. And, as a final indignity, men suffer erectile dysfunction—in other words, become impotent. And there is no cure for diabetes, it just has to be managed.

I have to say that at the end of Day One of definitive diagnosis I was not a happy Vegemite. Not normally given to depression (which in itself can raise blood sugar levels, as I found out later), Ros caught me gazing out the window with the corners of my mouth turned down, brooding about all the goodies I couldn't have any more, such as cakes, pastries, pies, soft and blue cheeses (which I love), fried fish and chips and, perhaps the most unkind cut of all, unmeasured libations of booze. There had been too much to take in on that first day and Ros sensibly suggested that I go back to Ron to hopefully hear some good news. And there was some.

The positives, according to my amiable GP, were that if I was a good lad and stuck to my low-fat, low-sugar diet, exercised and eased back on the grog, I'd be able to stave off most of the dire consequences perhaps for some years. I would, however, need to get my eyes and feet checked once a year, not to mention all the other blood and urine tests that were about to become part of my ongoing medical routine.

This sounded better, so I decided to push the envelope.

I put it to Ron with a great surge of optimism that if I stopped living in the unhealthy way I had been—I didn't think it had been all *that* evil—did all the recommended dieting and exercise, then maybe I'd live longer with diabetes than if I hadn't been diagnosed! Ron got a bit vague about that. That's another thing you learn quickly about diabetes. There's so much information that seems to be contradictory. Take for instance the confusion between Type 1 and Type 2 diabetes. Many of the books and information pamphlets available deal with both. As I was to discover, they are vastly different conditions—although they share many characteristics, particularly the complications.

Type 1 diabetes

Often in the past this condition was identified by the acronym IDDM (insulin dependent diabetes mellitus). It is the most common of the two diabetic conditions to affect young children and adults under 25. For reasons still being researched, the body's immune system destroys the insulin-producing cells of the pancreas—and there are often no obvious symptoms until 90 per cent of the insulin-producing cells are destroyed. Then the onset of symptoms happens very quickly.

In normal circumstances, insulin produced in the pancreas is used by the body to lower high sugar (glucose) levels in the blood, which naturally occur after eating a meal. Without insulin, blood glucose levels rise dramatically and the affected person quickly becomes ill. The symptoms are obvious and dramatic: a vicious cycle of excessive thirst and copious urination, lethargy and a general feeling of being unwell, blurred vision and other unpleasant side effects such as vomiting and an outbreak of monilia (thrush). The body's immune system is also affected, reducing the function of white cells to combat infection.

As the pancreas produces no insulin at all, those with Type 1 diabetes have to begin an insulin-injection regime immediately, and for life. Before the discovery of insulin, and how to produce it from animals, in 1922, Type 1 diabetes or IDDM was a death sentence for young people who developed it.

Type 2 diabetes

Type 2 diabetes, previously known as NIDDM (non-insulin dependent diabetes mellitus), often creeps up on people as there are no obvious symptoms in the early stages. Some people can have it for years before it gets picked up—often when a blood test is taken for a general health check-up, which is a good reason to have them, particularly in middle life and onward. Or symptoms become apparent, such as thirst, too frequent urination or blurred vision. If other family members have diabetes that's a good reason to get checked out as it can be inherited. Diagnosis is often confirmed by a glucose tolerance test, as I experienced, during which a heavily sugared drink is consumed after overnight fasting, and blood samples taken over a two hour period.

Unlike those with Type 1 diabetes, where the body produces no insulin at all, the pancreas of Type 2 (NIDDM) diabetics still produces insulin, but the insulin does not work properly, or there is not enough. A commonly used metaphor is that of a lock and a key. The insulin—a hormone—acts as a key to unlock the body's cells so that the sugar (glucose) can enter them. After glucose enters, the cells can immediately use it for energy, store it, or convert it to fat for later use as energy. As soon as the glucose leaves the blood and enters your cells, the glucose level falls. The pancreas cleverly notices this, and cuts back the release of insulin to prevent the glucose levels getting dangerously low. It's an amazing arrangement, and I'll return to it later in my own voyage of discovery around my newly diabetic body.

For some reason the lock gets rusty, and the insulin key doesn't enter efficiently. So glucose levels rise and stay too high.

At the same time the insulin producing cells in the pancreas seem to get weary and fail to produce enough insulin needed to get through the rusty lock.

If picked up early, many people with Type 2 diabetes—and I am one of them—can reduce their blood glucose to near normal levels through diet and exercise and losing excess weight. However, it is an incurable condition (at the moment) and as my GP, Ron, pointed out, it has to be managed. Even if I keep on the straight and narrow, eat a low-fat, low-sugar diet and get plenty of exercise, it is almost inevitable that, after a number of years (Ron couldn't be more specific because diabetes affects people in varying ways), I will probably have to go on some kind of oral medication to keep my glucose levels down. Ron thought it unlikely I would progress to injecting insulin, but some Type 2 patients do reach that stage.

Different types of diabetes

Type 1 diabetes—IDDM (insulin dependent diabetes mellitus)

- represents 10 to 15 per cent of all cases of diabetes
- occurs when the pancreas gland no longer produces the insulin needed
- is one of the most common chronic childhood diseases in developed nations
- is not caused by lifestyle factors.

Diagnosis

Usually in childhood or young adulthood, although it can occur at any age.

Symptoms

Usually abrupt onset and can include excessive thirst and urination, unexplained weight loss, weakness and fatigue, irritability.

Treatment

- lifelong daily insulin injections
- regular blood glucose level tests
- healthy eating plan
- regular physical activity.

Type 2 diabetes—NIDDM (non-insulin dependent diabetes mellitus)

- represents 85 to 90 per cent of all cases of diabetes
- occurs when the pancreas is not producing enough insulin and the insulin is not working effectively
- lifestyle factors such as unhealthy diet and lack of exercise can contribute to the development of Type 2 diabetes
- risk factors include family history.

Diagnosis

Usually in adults over the age of 45 but it is increasingly occurring at a younger age.

Symptoms

Sometimes symptoms go unnoticed as the disease develops gradually but they may include any of those for Type 1 diabetes plus blurred vision, skin infections, slow healing, tingling and numbness in the feet.

Treatment

Regular physical activity and healthy eating—over time treatment may progress from lifestyle modification to requiring tablets and/or insulin injections.

Gestational diabetes

- a form of diabetes that occurs in pregnancy (the mother does not have diabetes before pregnancy) and mostly disappears after the birth
- occurs in less than 9 per cent of pregnancies (it may be as high as 20 per cent amongst Aboriginal women and high-risk ethnic groups, including those from India, China, Asia and Pacific Islands)
- women over the age of 30, overweight, have a family history of Type 2 diabetes, had gestational diabetes during a previous pregnancy or have had difficulty bringing pregnancy to full term are at greater risk
- increases the risk of pregnancy complications
- significantly increases the risk for women to develop Type 2 diabetes later in life.

Pre-diabetes (insulin resistant)

Two million Australians have a condition known as pre-diabetes and if left untreated it may develop into Type 2 diabetes within five to ten years. Pre-diabetes is when blood glucose levels are higher than normal but not yet high enough for a diagnosis of Type 2 diabetes. In addition to the risk of developing diabetes, people with pre-diabetes are more likely to have a heart attack or stroke.

Courtesy of Diabetes Australia

I have to admit, for about a week after diagnosis I indulged in a certain amount of gloom and doom. Farewell to the indulgence of unrestricted eating and drinking. Let's face it, sex, eating and drinking are among life's greatest pleasures and as the advancing years necessarily diminished the former, the importance of the latter seemed to compensate most agreeably. But I won't draw that bow too long . . . Since those early days I've done more research, and my initial reaction was right on target for newly diagnosed Type 2s.

'This can't be happening to me. Why me anyway? What have I done to deserve this?' (Quite a lot actually but I'll leave that for the moment.) 'My life is going to be miserable from now on until I eventually cark it—probably because of bloody diabetes.'

I started to become aware of diabetic horror stories. A friend's parents were diabetic. Her mother had just died of kidney failure while her father was in hospital recuperating from having some of his toes amputated because of peripheral neuropathy (loss of sensation and bad circulation) caused, of course, by diabetes.

Fortunately I am a fairly optimistic person and not prone to dark moods for long. In any case my ex-nurse spouse, Ros, soon snapped me out of it. 'I mean, you haven't got cancer for heaven's sake. All you have to do is change your diet and lose some weight. You don't even have to give up grog, only cut back a bit, which will be good for you anyway! So snap out of it.'

Ros (who needed to shed a few kilos herself) decided to join me on the diabetic regime. In fact, if everyone ate like a diabetic should—low fat, low sugar and plenty of fruit and vegetables—we wouldn't have the public health problems that are clogging our hospitals with preventable diseases. (I'm starting to sound like a sanctimonious born-again wowser.) It certainly helps to have your partner travelling the same gastronomic road.

I snapped out of it.

It was quite extraordinary how many people I knew had diabetes. Some only revealed this after I'd mentioned my own diagnosis, like Bob, a New Zealand journalist friend who I've known for more than forty years. We worked on the same newspaper, briefly, in Hobart in 1960 and then shared a small house (with some other Australian journalists) in London shortly after that. I hadn't seen much of him since as he lives in Wellington and I've never been to New Zealand, other than an hour or so at Auckland International Airport when heading somewhere else. But we've kept in touch over the years. I was aware that Bob's wife Sarah had died in recent years. She also had diabetes, was obese and had undergone serious cardiac surgery. Bob wrote:

> Dear Tim,
>
> I'm very sorry to hear about the diabetes. But it's good to hear you can control it with diet.
>
> I'm not trying to lead you astray but I've had it for six years and, while following a reasonably good diet (using sugar extenders like Splenda), I've also been told to limit drinking to two glasses a day, and I tell the diabetes clinic with a straight face that by and large I stick to that (but the glass is a big one—about two wine glasses capacity—and when I'm out I sometimes stray to a bottle for me and whatever for the other folk).
>
> This has only given me the small stroke I had in March last year, high blood pressure, and a sore foot, so I figure I'm ahead so far. But even if it sort of works for me, everyone is

different and I don't necessarily recommend it to you. I shoot up with insulin and, like you, don't particularly enjoy the daily blood glucose tests.

My late wife Sarah used to challenge her diabetes head-on, which was unwise given that previously she had had a heart bypass operation. She used to whack 40 units of insulin in (a good dose) and then 'pig out' on chocolate, chocolate cake, chocolate biscuits, boiled sweets and, did I mention, chocolate? She figured she must be in a lot of credit with the insulin before balancing the books, as it were. It didn't work too well.

Tonight's menu will include lemon chicken, a particular potato dish, asparagus, tomatoes, mushrooms, a fairly standard sort of dessert (possibly low-fat ice cream and low-sugar fruit) and plenty of wine.

Enough of health. It's boring. Anyway, all you need to know for New Zealand is that the main dangers to health in this country are (a) our health system and (b) our doctors.

Yesterday I collected from the airport for my mother-in-law Sarah's slightly younger sister. On delivery, my mother-in-law said this was not her daughter but a balloon I'd found. Her daughter didn't mind, and said this was not her mother but her grandmother. Sarah's sister weighs 200 lb [90 kg], is 5 ft 4 in [162 cm] tall, has a big stomach and enormous breasts. While travelling in my little old car with her I couldn't help thinking—now this Honda is fitted with twin air bags.

Well, must go. If it's any comfort, you'll probably live for 20 more years and I hope the diabetes doesn't wholly run your life for that time.

Cheers,

Bob

I had a more reassuring email from Ken Chown, a television producer I'd worked with in Sydney in the 1970s. Ken, now retired, was diagnosed with Type 1 diabetes as a young man:

> Hi Tim
>
> Yes, it's not the best news about the diabetes. I have now had it for more than 40 years and, although I get fed up with the testing routine (as essential as the diet and exercise), at seventy-one I feel fit and well. I could be slowing down but I enjoy doing most things.
>
> You and I have different types of diabetes. Mine is Type 1, which used to be described as juvenile onset diabetes (although I was 30 when I was diagnosed), and yours is Type 2, which is the more common form and where it's determined that the pancreas may still be functioning but not to optimum levels. Diet and possibly oral medication are usually sufficient.
>
> But the diet is a very good healthy diet—low in fat and low in sugar. The only 'diabetic' foods I touch are diet jellies because I like jelly and they bulk out the fruit. Two or three fresh peaches will give me six serves. I am a yoghurt enthusiast and I have plain or fat-reduced yoghurt once or twice a day. No ice cream and rarely cream. I also ignore all jams and marmalades even if they are 100 per cent fruit.
>
> Most diabetic diets today are prescribed to cut down on the fat and added sugar; it may take some time to get used to this regime but you will be feeling progressively better—a wonderful feeling. Sadly, though, there will be a routine, which can be a pain in the butt.
>
> I have also heard the alcohol restriction but both my GP and my specialist know that I drink and enjoy it. There is little sugar in red wine and, anyway, we have to watch our alcohol

content if we're out or going somewhere. I have occasional alcohol-free days—if I am taking someone to the airport, or attending some important meeting.

Good luck with it all, Tim. I'd like to know how it goes. And Diabetes Australia does a fabulous job in managing the Diabetes Scheme (which gives us cheap needles and sensor strips, although the tab is picked up by the Commonwealth Government).

I'll keep in touch.

Cheers (you'll need it),

Ken

Although Ken was Type 1 and Barry Type 2, I thought he might be a better role model. Then there was Kim Boyer, a fellow Tasmanian, who was working at the time as a senior health bureaucrat. Like me, she was only recently diagnosed.

Hi Tim

Well, what a surprise. The finger pricking bit gets easier, I can assure you. In the first month I had heaps of hassles but now I'm a dab hand.

What I find hard in the diet stakes is the severe rationing/elimination of foods that are full of fat which I previously thought were healthy. Like good cheeses, especially. Also quiches, veggie pastries and pies, samosas and pakoras. And no gin and tonic before dinner or when playing Scrabble.

Eating out is a pain because a lot of the challenge is in how stuff is cooked, the sauces and so on. In fact, when I leave work in a few months I am going to write a guide to Tassie dining from a diabetic perspective, because there are few quality restaurants that provide exciting food which is genuinely healthy.

I have given up baked veggies, all butter and cream (apart

from low-fat stuff), chocolates, sweet biscuits, etc. No added salt and no tinned food with high-salt content.

Am eating heaps more fruit, vegetables and carbohydrates and far less meat and eggs, having a decent breakfast, no between meal snacks, and, until dinner time, have only water or the odd skinny coffee or herb tea.

I've negotiated four standard glasses of vino providing I have no other naughty things—and every so often the standard becomes larger than life. I call it Kim's standard!! This seems to work. With two pills a day I stay in the 5s and 6s (within normal blood glucose range) but there is a big jump with silly little things like chicken wings or small slivers of goat's cheese! Also I exercise heaps more, have lost 10 to 12 kg and generally feel miles better—less tired and crabby!

But every so often I have bouts of sleeplessness and depression which, having a physical reason for them, make them easier to deal with.

The educator, diet and podiatrist people here are great and I also have a spiffy specialist (a young woman) who is really helpful as my blood pressure has been massive and she is prepared to try to work out a range of possible solutions that aren't all drug based.

So it gives you a huge shock, but it is manageable. Ros may like to talk to Fred about how he has changed his cooking style and how he copes with me being moody every so often!

Hope that helps!

Love,

Kim

I wasn't sure how long Kim had had diabetes before being diagnosed, but probably for a few years because she had to go straight on to medication and was finding her diabetic management initially tricky. It was certainly helpful to share information with friends who also had diabetes, and mostly reassuring.

My first priority was to shed at least ten kilos, because carrying extra fat makes it difficult for the body to process the insulin that was mercifully still being produced in my embattled pancreas—not an organ of my body I'd ever given much thought to I must say. As a journalist, I had thought my liver might be the first major organ to be threatened. As it happened the poor thing was a bit stressed, but was about to get a comparative rest. Let's face it, I knew I was carrying too much weight. I have done so for at least the past 20 years, probably more. But the time to get serious about losing some of it never seemed to arrive. Now everyone kept telling me that excess fat was bad, bad news for people with diabetes.

I have to say that being told you have an incurable condition which has to be managed sensibly or your health will be seriously affected, concentrates the mind wonderfully. It is often said that the most difficult part of any diet is to stick to it. I wanted to start as I meant to keep on—eating the right food, smaller portions, and combining that with (shock horror) only two or three glasses of wine a day. To do that I didn't want to have to count calories or think about it all the time. Just find out what I could eat, and get on with it. I figured there would be two phases of this—actually losing the weight, and then the maintenance of that weight loss, which might hopefully involve less of a hair-shirt regime.

The time to start was now.

CHAPTER TWO

Facing up to it

I have to admit to not being a group person. I am easily bored. My fledgling career in ABC program management was fatally eroded by an inability to take meetings seriously and an uncontrollable urge to make flippant or smart-arse remarks. But I did need information on Type 2 diabetes urgently, particularly how to begin managing it. So when my GP, Ron, suggested I go to the next group session conducted by the local area health service at Forster, I did so with mixed feelings.

While no-one wants to get diabetes, there are worse places to get it. The twin coastal towns of Forster and Tuncurry are in dead-set retirement belt territory. There is even a retirement home called 'Golden Ponds'. So many older Australians live here that our local Woolworths and Coles have to charter extra semi-trailers each week just to keep their shelves stocked with enough blue rinse. One of the results of this is that there are excellent diabetes services available, as I was about to discover.

Ros very kindly offered to come with me to the group session at the Forster Community Health Centre. Our group of 17 people (including some other valiant spouses) were all over 65, pretty evenly balanced between men and women, except that while some of the women were overweight, just about all of the blokes were hefting around far too much flesh, including some classic 'Norm' beer bellies. We were all recently diagnosed, although Phyllis had come back for a top-up of information on what she should be doing.

When we got around to talking about exercise, Phyllis, who was still an ample woman, said she had been over 100 kilos when diagnosed, but had trimmed off 25 of those through a combination of diet and line dancing. I muttered to my partner that I'd rather clamber into the pine box and start staring permanently up at the lid right now than do line dancing. Ros hissed in my ear to behave myself.

Our group session was addressed by the health centre diabetes nurse educator, Ivy Semple, a very caring, well-informed woman who steered us through the basics of diabetes, reminding us that it was a life-long condition with no cure which would have to be managed by healthy eating habits, exercise, perhaps medication and a positive attitude. Smoking, bad for us anyway, was even more so for diabetics who were prone to blood vessel blockages. 'Is anyone here a smoker?' she asked.

'Yes please', said 75-year-old Noel, who told the group he had been diagnosed for ten days, fourteen hours and six minutes.

We were also given the basics of a good healthy diet by John Jones, the area dietitian, who explained why diabetics needed to monitor their carbohydrate intake throughout the day, hopefully with foods with a low glycaemic index (GI),[1] and avoid saturated fats like the plague. We began to learn how to read food labels for their nutrition, fat and sugar content, to cut through the jargon. 'Now, let's take someone at random and find out what you had for lunch yesterday', said John cheerfully.

'Fish and chips', said big Russell. 'And they were bloody beautiful.'

John blanched and found someone who had nibbled at a wholegrain salad sandwich, washed down with tomato juice followed by an apple. Ivy had very kindly prepared some diabetically friendly cakes and biscuits for morning tea, but Russell was so shaken by the detail of the kind of diet that was supposed to replace his breakfast of fried eggs and bacon, a dog's eye and dead horse for lunch, and half a dozen skewies of beer before his evening steak and chips, that he eschewed the apricot slices made without butter, and told me he was heading outside for an urgently needed ciggie.

At question time, one of the thinner diabetic blokes present, Kev, asked whether home-brewed beer was better for people with diabetes. Now I have always believed my late father had it right when he said, 'Home brewed beer is like farting. Your own seems all right.' John looked bemused and said it depended how strong it was. Kev, who had seemed gloomy from the start, looked positively suicidal when he heard that.

---

1 The glycaemic index (GI) of a food is determined by measuring how much the actual rise in blood glucose levels is after eating a particular food and comparing that figure to the effect of eating pure glucose. This provides a ranking of foods. Glucose has a ranking of 100 and most other carbohydrate foods are ranked underneath this figure. A fuller explanation, with examples of food with a low GI, can be found in chapter six, 'What can I eat?'.

At this point I should say most newly diagnosed diabetics in the room were taking all this extremely seriously. As I had found with some of my own friends, though, quite a few of the overweight men seemed to be in almost total denial. The women present were unfailingly attentive to what was being said and the importance of maintaining their diet and exercise regimes.

Our lecturers were certainly putting a positive spin on things. Perhaps that was deliberate at this point in our diabetic education. Stress by itself, we learned, can raise your blood glucose levels. Then we were told about the importance of regular eye checks. People with diabetes may develop retinopathy, where small blood vessels are damaged at the back of the eye which may result in loss of vision. Ivy told us that if damage was found, it could be stabilised by laser treatment. We were told it was also advisable to get our feet checked by a podiatrist at least once a year to check on a condition called diabetic neuropathy, which could result in numbness, pins and needles, or unexplained pain—leading to more serious consequences if not treated. I suppose the good news for the recently diagnosed like me is that these problems tend to occur in people who have had undiagnosed diabetes for some years.

Towards the end of the session I noticed a short, very circumferentially challenged man in tailored shorts take a seat at the back of the room. Ross was the President of the local branch of Diabetes Australia, which he wanted us to join as he explained when he came forward to speak to us. Ross told us that he used to be well over 100 kilos but had lost 20 since being diagnosed. He was an enthusiastic, cheerful bloke who outlined what Diabetes Australia did—organising cheaper testing equipment and other diabetic gear was one benefit, as well as fund raising for diabetic research, with a particular emphasis on the plight of children with Type 1 who had to inject insulin up to four times a day. He was so upbeat about the social joys of belonging to the local Diabetes Australia branch that I started to feel sorry for non-diabetics who failed to qualify.

One thing he emphasised was that Diabetes Australia was a life-line of good information and a conduit to cheaper products for people with diabetes. I immediately signed up for both Diabetes Australia and the National Diabetes Services Scheme (funded by the Federal Government and administered by Diabetes Australia), and was soon very glad I had done so.

Join Diabetes Australia and NDSS

The next steps after being diagnosed with diabetes should be:

1 join Diabetes Australia
2 complete the NDSS registration form and have your doctor sign it
3 get to know your diabetes team—make an appointment to see a dietitian and a diabetes educator—and the team includes your doctor, eye specialist, pharmacist, and podiatrist.

Diabetes Australia is a non-government, community-based, donor-supported charity dedicated to caring for all people with diabetes. To contact them ring 1300 136 588 from anywhere in Australia and you will be connected to your state branch.

It is recommended that people with diabetes carry their current Diabetes Australia membership card and their white NDSS registration card with them at all times.

Each card means different things and gives important but different benefits to the holder. Registration with NDSS does not automatically

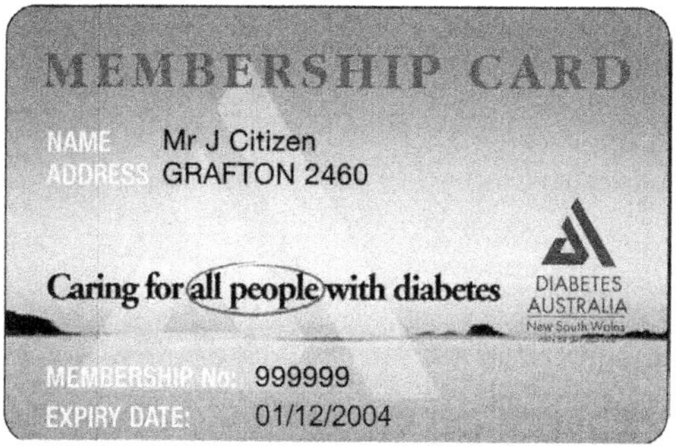

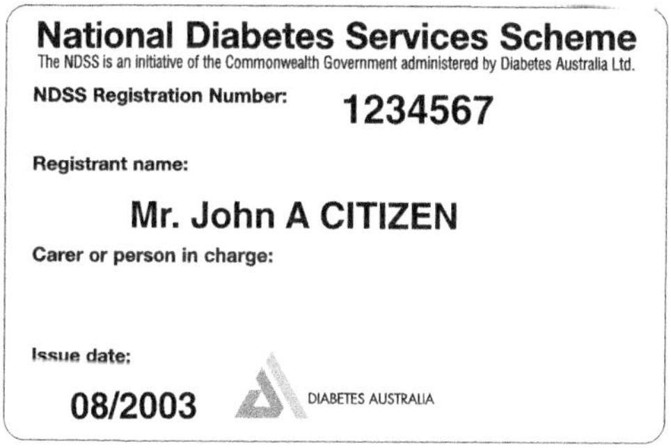

imply membership of Diabetes Australia and vice versa. Diabetes Australia branches will answer any questions about the use of these cards.

Reasons to join

The National Diabetes Services Scheme (NDSS) card recognises the holder is registered with the scheme as a person with diabetes. The NDSS card entitles the bearer to free syringes and pen needles and test strips at subsidised prices. This national service scheme was established following considerable lobbying by Diabetes Australia. The government has since appointed Diabetes Australia to administer the scheme on its behalf. That is why the DA brand appears on the registration card.

Diabetes Australia–NSW is the third oldest diabetes organisation in the world, and has been serving people with diabetes for over 60 years. Membership opens the door to many unique services and benefits available only to holders of a current membership card. In NSW, dietitians, educators and other health professionals are available to answer telephone queries about diabetes management, diet and any other areas of concern that may arise. This is a free service to members.

Other membership advantages include a free national magazine and state magazine every quarter, which includes updates on research and the latest news and information on developments in medical advances, trends in diabetes management, and general health care.

The membership is free for the first year to all people 18 and under. There are special supervised, informative and fun children's camps.

There is also free membership to a local branch or support group, whichever a member chooses to join. These peer groups provide support and information through regular meetings.

Diabetes Australia members can access exclusive areas of a website at www.diabetesnsw.com.au for up-to-the-minute information on managing diabetes, the latest news on research and advances in management from around the world, and the ability to talk to Diabetes Australia experts.

There was a bewildering amount of information to take in at my first Forster Community Health Centre session, but it was made very clear that carrying excess weight was bad news for those of us with diabetes. My GP, Ron, had also explained to me that he couldn't really assess whether my condition could be diet and exercise controlled or whether I would have to take medication until I had lost some weight and been on an appropriate diet for at least three months.

Now I was well aware that I was a fairly porky person and I used to say things like, 'Well a man needs to carry a bit of bulk in later life', as though it was akin to a camel's hump which would save me in times of famine. But the famine never came. With losing weight a key part of good management, it seemed sensible to get on with it. I needed to shed at least ten kilos, to bring me back from 85 to 75 kilograms.

As I've said previously, I didn't want to be thinking about food and diet all the time. I wanted to get into an eating routine that would do the job fairly quickly and not leave me without energy, feeling sorry for myself. When I'd reached my target weight, I decided, I would be able to take off the hair shirt to some extent and find out a bit more about what goodies I *could* eat when I'd reached what the diet experts called the 'maintenance' stage—the time when most dieters put all that lost weight back on again.

I figured the best thing to do was to adapt what I normally eat to the new regime, and try to stick to that. Any tendency to stray from the path of virtue would not only be frowned on by my ex-nurse partner, but was also tempered by a certain amount of raw fear in me that my quality of life would deteriorate in the years ahead.

I did manage to shed 10 kilos in three months, and this is how I did it.

Tim's diabetically friendly weight-loss diet

Breakfast was easy. It was summer when I started and all I ate for breakfast was un-toasted muesli (avoid the ones with coconut, which has naughty saturated fats) with a generous spoonful of psyllium husks (good for daily regularity and to guard against bowel cancer), some tinned apricots with no added sugar, and a generous dollop of low-fat fruit yoghurt. Just that, and a cuppa—with artificial sweeteners of course, and a dash of low-fat milk.

Nothing for morning tea. People with Type 1 diabetes have to make sure they have regular intakes of carbohydrate throughout the day, but those with Type 2 generally don't have to snack between meals (unless they are taking certain tablets).

What I had for lunch depended on whether Ros made it, or I did. I've never been a great fan of iceberg lettuce, which I've always associated with those tired pub salads featuring lettuce with brown edges, limp slices of tomato and raw onion rings. But sometimes a man has to do what he has to do. Ros—who keeps making the point that she didn't marry me to do lunches—cuts up some crisp iceberg lettuce, adds some three-bean mix, perhaps some anchovies, chopped up salad veggies such as tomato, cucumber or avocado, maybe some tinned corn topped with a dollop of cottage cheese, and a small dash of low-fat salad dressing. This is accompanied by two corn biscuits. The first time I munched through all this I felt like a rabbit, but I have to confess I've come to like it as time has gone on. (This may be partly connected to the reality that I don't have to make it.) This is washed down with a diet Coke (that does no harm but isn't wildly healthy either), and lunch ends with two pieces of fruit, an apple or pear, or a banana or mandarin.

If I get my own lunch I get two slices of wholegrain Bürgen bread with a smear of polyunsaturated margarine, a few slices of ham off-the-bone (processed fat-impregnated luncheon meats are to be avoided) seasoned with hot English mustard or a smear of fruit chutney and tomato. A minor indulgence is a Vita-Weat biscuit with a thin slice of matured cheddar cheese (low-fat cheese is not only tasteless but stacked full of sodium to try and make it taste better, so you might as well have a smidgeon of the real thing) and the equivalent of a teaspoon of honey. It's a great combination, and honey (and sugar in general) isn't the great bogey that people with diabetes once thought it was, so long as you don't pig out on the stuff. Diet Coke, and two pieces of fruit.

No afternoon snack.

Before dealing with dinner, I must address the all-important regime of booze. In my declining years I had stopped drinking alcohol at lunch time anyway (with the exception of an occasional old-fashioned boozy lunch, generally with old journalist mates), but our normal evening regime started with nibbles and a beer, followed by anything up to four glasses of wine, sometimes five—and even more if we were out socialising or having friends to dinner. Let's face it, I didn't count glasses anyway at such times. The idea of alcohol-free days seemed too horrible to contemplate at this time of general diabetic deprivation, so I decided to adopt a regime of no more than three glasses of wine in the evening—and maybe only one or two during the weight-loss phase.

As a way of delaying the urge to fall heavily down the neck of a nice bottle of wine too quickly, I was alerted (by a fellow Type 2 I met at the Health Centre) to a splendid brand of low-joule ginger beer which he swore by. I tried it and liked it a lot. It was less sweet than sugared ginger beer, and absolutely full flavoured. I would challenge anyone to pick the difference. It's so good I'll give them a commercial—Saxbys Diet Ginger Beer. So I adopted a new regime (which I'm still happy with a year on from diagnosis) of having a ginger beer when 6 p.m. arrived and those pesky brain synapses started screaming, 'time for a drink, time for a drink'. While Ros enjoyed her usual beer (I forgave her for this) I drank my ginger beer as we toyed with a few suitable nibbles.

Ros found a brilliant way of splitting pita bread, sprinkling it with lemon pepper, and crisping it in the oven. That went well with some kalamata olives and reduced-fat fetta cheese and—the *real* discovery, passed on by a friend, Nina—almonds microwaved and sprinkled with a little soy sauce (the recipe is below). These are sensational, much better than scorched almonds in my view. Nuts, I had already learned from John Jones, the dietitian, were brilliant for diabetics, containing mono-unsaturated oil that actually added years to your life. I'm exaggerating of course, but nuts are excellent fodder for Type 1 and Type 2 diabetics. So this is a nutritious treat for everyone really.

Nina's nuts

Buy a big bag of raw almonds from the supermarket. They are not expensive. Get a Pyrex dish (I use a shallow casserole lid about 24 centimetres in diameter) and cover the bottom with a layer of the almonds. You will need to experiment with the power of your microwave, but I put ours on high for two minutes. Then stir the almonds about a bit, and microwave for another three minutes. If they start to go brown they are burning, so cut back on the cooking time. However, they need to be good and hot because when you take them out, you sprinkle them with some light Asian soy, which foams and bubbles when it hits the hot nuts. Scramble the nuts around in the soy until all the almonds are coated and the soy absorbed. Then tip them out onto a piece of paper towel to cool, before storing in an airtight container. If you do more than one batch at a time you may need to reduce the microwave time by a minute, sometimes more, as the Pyrex dish will gradually get hotter. It is a good idea to give them a stir around after the first three minutes. Believe me, once you have mastered preparing almonds in this way you will be addicted for life!

Before leaving the pre-dinner nibbles suggestions (and, remember, these must not be overdone in the weight-loss phase of a diet), we sometimes just get a piece of raw salmon, cut it into bite-sized pieces as sashimi, and dip the pieces into soy and wasabi. Just that . . . nothing else. Fish of almost any kind is good news for everyone, particularly those with diabetes, because of its utterly admirable omega-3 polyunsaturated fats.

I suppose the biggest trap of the evening meal is to eat portions that are too large. Simply cutting back on quantity is an efficient way to diet. Most of us eat too much anyway, mostly because it feels good at the time.

Grilled steak with all the fat removed or grilled fish and vegetables are excellent fodder. Curiously enough, potatoes have a high glycaemic index (GI), so they can only be taken in moderation. Rice is not good news either for this reason, but some varieties, such as basmati, have a lower GI (meaning, this form of carbohydrate is absorbed by the body more slowly). Sweet potato and the yam family of vegetables have a low GI, and so does corn. Ros has experimented with polenta instead of mashed potato, which we find very palatable.

A stir-fry using lean chicken, pork, lamb and beef, mixed in with plenty of vegetables, in a non-stick wok with just a spray of virgin olive oil is a favourite of ours. I'm particularly fond of vegetable curries, in fact Indian, Thai and Malaysian curries of all kinds. Ros even manages an occasional laksa using light coconut milk. (We have since been told by an Indian friend that light and creamy Carnation milk is an excellent substitute for coconut milk.) The main aim is to eat plenty of vegetables and some lean meat for protein.

And dinner is the time when I enjoy my two (or three) glasses of red wine. It is better to eat while drinking alcohol, so this is a happy situation for me and almost 'best' diet practice. (Okay, I'm kidding myself, but if I can't have a glass or two of red I'll have to reassess the future of life on this planet.) During the weight-loss phase I tried (and generally succeeded) in keeping my wine intake to two glasses a night—occasionally only one.

A small dollop of low-fat ice-cream and some fruit rounded out the evening meal.

Summary of Tim's weight-loss diet

Breakfast

- glass of tomato juice
- muesli with low-fat milk, low-fat fruit yoghurt, tinned apricots and a heaped tablespoon of psyllium husks
- tea with a dash of low-fat milk and artificial sweeteners

Lunch

- mixed lettuce salad with cottage cheese, low-fat salad dressing
- two 'corn thins' biscuits
- diet Coke
- Vita-Weat biscuit with thin slice of mature cheddar cheese and smear of honey
- two pieces of fruit

or

- sandwich of two slices of wholegrain Burgen bread with a smear of margarine
- sliced ham and English mustard
- sliced tomato
- diet Coke
- two pieces of fruit

Dinner

- modest starter nibbles of low-fat fetta, kalamata olives and microwaved almonds (see above recipe)
- pita bread split and crisped in oven with lemon pepper
- low-joule Saxby ginger beer
- stir-fry of vegetables with lean chicken, beef or pork cooked in a non-stick wok with minimum virgin olive oil and steamed basmati rice

or

- grilled fish with sweet potato, pumpkin, broccoli and carrots (or other veg)

or

- vegetable curry (with a little light coconut milk as an indulgence) and basmati rice

or

- pasta (low GI) with a tomato and pesto sauce

or

- grilled lean steak with English mustard, polenta (instead of potato) and steamed veggies

or

- lean chicken (without skin) grilled in tikka and yoghurt marinade, with polenta (or sweet potato) and steamed veggies
- small serve of low-fat ice-cream (or Vitari) with unsweetened tinned fruit
- herbal tea (sometimes)

Tim's exercise regime

It was made very clear to me during the first sessions I had at the Community Health Centre in Forster that regular exercise not only played a vital role in controlling diabetes, but was essential in the weight-losing phase as well. Exercise, as most people know, burns up energy, including those reserves of excess fat that our primeval survival instinct has been storing against that possible famine (well, I have to put a positive spin on that) and it is also very important in lowering blood glucose levels.

Having, many years ago, bought one of those stationary exercise bicycles, to only throw it out after using it just three times, I knew not to ride down that sterile road again. I'm also not a gym person, nor is there one near where I live. I'm too old to jog—and it's bad for your knees anyway. (Whenever anyone of mature years jogs past me I usually say in a loud voice, 'No good will come of this you know'.) And being brought up in Tasmania I'm a hopeless swimmer, flailing along with my head out of the water and absolutely unable to swim laps in that graceful way just about every other Australian seems to have built in to them—so that was out as well. I pondered what to do.

Vigorous walking is one of the best exercises—kind to the knees, and it can be built into the daily routine, which is an important factor in exercising regularly. So, weather permitting, I set off at 7 a.m. to walk along the back of Boomerang Beach, where I live, and over a hill to our local shops to buy the morning paper. It's about a five kilometre round trip and takes 45 minutes. (They say you should try and exercise for at least 40 minutes in one go to get the most benefit.) At the same time I get to listen to the ABC Radio National breakfast program (of course!), including the news and *AM*, via my trusty portable radio. It's also a great way of keeping in touch with your surroundings and some of its inhabitants. Living in a small community like ours, people actually make eye contact and smile when they pass each other on these morning perambulations. Quite often I see dolphins slicing through the clear windows of a wave just before it breaks into a smother of foam. They are clearly doing it just for fun, like the early morning surfers—some of them the local 'tradies' from building sites.

I try to do this early morning walk six times a week. (The Sunday papers are so crappy I can't be bothered to walk for them.) In addition, I also got a bicycle—a moving one—and I try and ride my bicycle to the local post office (a 45 minute round trip) to get the mail at least three or four times a week. For the rest of the time I seem to sit in front of my computer and write, which is probably one of the factors that brought on my Type 2 diabetes. I wish I'd exercised more assiduously in years past—but it's no good thinking that now.

Much to my surprise (and pleasure) the kilos started dropping away. I managed to shed my ten kilos in three months, despite a break in routine during a three-week journey to Antarctica where shipboard life makes you ravenous, and self control has to be worked on. I had to get my pants taken in, and extra notches gauged in to my fat-man's belts. The important thing about exercise is to find out what suits you, be it walking, cycling, swimming, underwater aerobics, line dancing, skipping, tennis or farnarkling (apologies to John Clarke), and just keep doing it regularly.

Did it work for me?

At the end of my first three months since diagnosis with Type 2 diabetes I was due for an important and defining test which would assess how I was managing my diabetes, and whether I could do so with diet and exercise alone, or whether I would have to have daily medication to keep my blood glucose levels within bounds. It is called the HbA1c test (otherwise known as glycosylated haemoglobin test) and is something everyone with diabetes should know about and understand why it is important.

This test needs to be done regularly—usually every three months, although some GPs may order it every six months.

During those first three months, I had been pricking the sides of my fingers twice a day and recording my blood glucose levels in the diary that comes with the testing machine. To get the profile my GP needed, he asked me to test at different times on alternate days. The first day I tested before breakfast, and two hours after lunch. The second day, two hours after breakfast and two hours after the evening meal. People without diabetes generally have blood glucose levels between 4 to 8 mmol/L. 'Ideal control' is from 4 to 6 mmol/L before meals, and up to 8 mmol/L two hours after meals. 'Satisfactory control' for people with Type 2 diabetes is from 6 to 7 mmol/L before meals, and less than or equal to 11 mmol/L two hours after meals. Higher levels than this are, of course, considered unsatisfactory.

Looking back at my slightly bloodstained diary records for those first few months (my finger pricking skills developed over time) I now see that I wasn't doing too badly, with readings ranging mainly from fives to sevens, with the occasional eight or some nines. Doctor Ron had wanted to know the bad news—in other words, I had to test after indulgence, rather than waiting for a goody goody meal to make my BGL (blood glucose level) entry. Even if I had cooked the books, the all-important HbA1c test would reveal all.

Red blood cells conveniently live for 120 days. So they provide a record of the level of glucose attached to those cells over that time. The test would also provide an indication of where I was in my on-going battle with diabetes, by calculating a percentage. In broad brush terms, anything below 7 per cent (and above 5 per cent) would be good news. Over 7 per cent would mean

I would be looking towards medication to lower my blood sugars, or even moving to injecting insulin.

Doctor Ron also ordered a fasting blood test to see how my cholesterol levels were (and how my valiant liver was bearing up to its reduced red wine intake), as well as a battery of other biological barometers. In addition I had to provide a urine sample, collected during the night before the HbA1c test, to see if my kidneys were functioning adequately. (It is possible to lose up to 90 per cent of kidney function without any obvious symptoms!)

Ron told me that research in the United Kingdom had shown that people with diabetes registering 7 per cent on the HbA1c test, and who then managed to reduce that by even 1 per cent but hopefully more, had won themselves enormous benefits, lessening the likelihood of the side effects of diabetes, such as heart disease, strokes, peripheral nerve damage, impaired kidney function and diabetic retinopathy (eye damage). So it was with more than average interest that I awaited the results of my first HbA1c once-over.

To my delight, it was 5.6 per cent—actually within the 'normal' range. Ron said I had been doing well with my diabetes control, but cautioned against being too cocky. I would need to keep working at keeping my diabetes at bay, and these were early days.

Still, it wasn't a bad start! I cracked a half-way decent bottle of red that night with Ros to mark the occasion.

CHAPTER THREE

Why ants like your urine

I'm pleased for Ron, my GP, that he didn't have to diagnose me in the seventeenth century, when doctors could only recognise diabetes by tasting the urine of their patients to see if it was sweet. Not that they could do much for their patients after this heroic act because, although they could recognise the symptoms of diabetes, it was not known what caused it, and treatment was idiosyncratic and generally ineffective. As late as 1850 a French physician advised his diabetic patients to eat extra large quantities of sugar!

The term diabetes was coined by the Greek physician Arataeus of Cappadocia (now a region of Turkey) in AD 150 to describe the excessive flow, or 'siphoning', of urine that was such a dramatic symptom of the disease. He had a vivid turn of phrase when describing diabetes:

> . . . being a melting down of the flesh and limbs into urine. Its cause is of a cold and humid nature as in dropsy. The course is a common one, namely the kidneys and bladder; for the patients never stop making water, but the flow is incessant, as if from the opening of aqueducts. The nature of the disease then is chronic . . . the patient is short-lived if the constitution of the disease is completely established; for the melting is rapid, the death speedy . . . life is disgusting and painful; thirst unquenchable . . .

Arataeus was, of course, describing the drastic consequences of Type 1 diabetes. Type 2 was not recognised as a separate condition until the mid-twentieth century.

Diabetes, although not named as such, was also recognised by Egyptian physicians some 3500 years ago. A document known as the Ebers Papyrus, around 1552 BC, detailed remedies for the passing of too much urine. The Egyptian doctors recommended that those affected with the malady go on a diet of bear, fruits, grains and honey, which was reputed to stifle the excessive urination.

The connection between diabetes and sugar is often noted historically. Dr D. A. Pyke of King's College Hospital in London, wrote that, 'perhaps the ants deserve the credit for discovering the sweetness of diabetic urine'.[1] Indian scholars in the fourth century BC described the clinical features of diabetes and noted that ants clustered around the urine of diabetics. Similar observations about sweet urine were made in China in the seventh century AD by Chen Chhuan, and later by Avicenna, an Arab physician of the eleventh century. An English physician,

---

1 *Preamble: The History of Diabetes.*

Thomas Willis, rediscovered the sweetness of diabetic urine in 1674 and was the first to use the Latin word *mellitus* (honeyed). A hundred years later another English doctor, Matthew Dobson, also identified sugar in the urine of diabetics, but he also made the crucial observation of an excess of sugar in the blood.

Diabetes was rampant during the fifteenth, sixteenth and seventeenth centuries, the era when doctors had the unenviable task of tasting the urine of their patients. Accounts of the diets of the middle class in northern European countries during that time detail meals of many courses of roast meats, dripping with fat, rich and sugary pastries and plenty of butter and cream, with little coarse red or green leafy vegetables. Two schools of thought then emerged. One school believed in replacing the sugar lost in the urine, and the other thought it best to restrict the intake of carbohydrates. Thomas Willis recommended a diet limited to milk, barley water and bread—high in carbohydrates but low in calories. A century later some doctors urged a high-fat, high-protein and low-carbohydrate diet, pre-dating the controversial Dr Atkins, of mainly meat and fat. None of the physicians of those times knew what they were treating, and they believed diabetes was a disease of the blood, kidneys, liver or stomach or a combination of the lot. Eating as little as possible seems to have been the most effective therapy—the French physician Bouchardat wrote that the limited availability of food in Paris during the Franco–Prussian war of 1870–71 caused a reduction in sugar in the urine of his diabetic patients.

Medical scientists slowly homed in on what might be causing diabetes. The liver remained the chief suspect, then in the nineteenth century, scientist and medico, Frenchman Claude Bernard, discovered that the liver stored glycogen and secreted a sugary substance into the blood. He assumed an excess of this secretion caused diabetes.

The pancreas was known to produce digestive juices, but the clumps of ductless cells in the pancreas were thought to be unrelated to this function. The ductless cells were identified by a Strasbourg medical student, Paul Langerhans, in 1867. He called these three types of cells alpha, beta and delta. They are scattered throughout the pancreas, 'like currents in a pudding'—a commonly used metaphor. These little islands of tissue were quite different in appearance from the rest of the gland, but were not connected to any ducts, so it seemed reasonable to suppose that their secretion, whatever it was, went straight into the circulation. In fact, the wondrously named Islets of Langerhans, as they became known, produce the all-important insulin yet to be isolated and identified.

Twenty-two years later, in 1879, the discovery that removing the pancreas caused diabetes was finally made by chance—as are many pivotal medical discoveries. Dr Pyke described this milestone as such:

> Von Mering, a German physician in Strasburg, was interested in digestion. He wanted to know what role the pancreas played. He wanted to try the effect of removing it but thought that this was impossible. His colleague, Oscar Minkowski, said, 'Bah, I can take out the pancreas'. He could and he did. Then the unexpected happened. The next day the laboratory technician complained that the dog was urinating all over the cage, in spite of having been house-trained. Minkowski realised at once what this might mean, tested the urine and found glucose. He had produced diabetes by removing the pancreas, therefore the pancreas contained an antidiabetic substance.

Von Mering was only mildly interested; the rest of the story is Minkowski's.

Minkowski knew he was on to something, but he and his researchers were not able to extract or identify the antidiabetic substance from the pancreas, neither could many other workers in Europe and North America. They all knew what was at stake. It was thought that the pancreas was producing a secretion which regulated the metabolism of carbohydrates. The Islets of Langerhans were the chief suspects, but the secretion still eluded isolation and identification.

The breakthrough had to wait until the twentieth century. In 1921, in Canada, Frederick Banting was an unsuccessful orthopaedic surgeon ('in itself something of a rarity', commented the distinguished historian on diabetes, Dr Pyke) who had read about the association between the destruction of the pancreas and diabetes. He decided to find out why, but curiously did not investigate other experimental work in this area. Pyke thinks that this was his strength. 'He didn't know how difficult the problem was. Nothing would stop him.'

The Professor of Physiology at the University of Toronto, J. J. R. Macleod, gave Dr Banting laboratory space, a research assistant, a medical student, Charles Best, and ten dogs on which to experiment for eight weeks. Their first efforts were unsuccessful, but late in 1921 Banting and Best succeeded in extracting a relatively pure islet secretion which they injected into a dog whose pancreas had been removed. Its blood sugar was lowered immediately, and the dog was saved. Further injections confirmed their initial good results. At last it seemed that, if diabetes could not be cured, it could at least be controlled. The researchers managed to extract sufficient quantities of 'isletin', as they called the extract, from cattle to sustain their experiments.

The extract from the Islets of Langerhans in the pancreas of animals had to be made suitable for human use. Banting and Best turned to James B. Collip, Professor of Biochemistry at the University of Alberta, to help achieve this. Banting and Best heroically used the purified extract on themselves to test for adverse reactions, and then on 11 January 1922, 14-year-old Leonard Thompson achieved his place in medical history by being the first patient to receive insulin. He had had Type 1 diabetes for two years, and the insulin undoubtedly saved his life. Photographs taken before and after his first four months of treatment show a skeletal, very ill boy transformed into a healthy looking teenager who had gained 19 pounds (8.6 kg) in that time.

Collip and Best applied to patent the extraction method, and generously assigned the patent to the University of Toronto. They planned to call the extracted secretion *isletin* but this was changed to *insulin* after the work of a French researcher in 1909, J. de Meyer, who had first used the term—*insula* being Latin for island—because of its suspected connection with the Islets of Langerhans.

Many researchers had contributed to the discovery of insulin, but the Nobel Prize for Physiology and Medicine was awarded jointly to Dr Banting and Professor Macleod. Showing great generosity of spirit, Banting gave half his share of the prize to Charles Best, and Macleod did the same for James Collip.

Until insulin was isolated and able to be injected into Type 1 diabetes sufferers in 1922, the only possible outcome was a slow and lingering death. In her history to celebrate sixty years since the founding of Diabetes Australia–New South Wales, *And Not to Yield: Sixty Years On, 1937–1997*, author Margaret Molloy quotes from the memories of Dr John Kempson Maddox, who was a fourth year medical student at the University of Sydney in 1922. (Dr Kempson Maddox was a principal figure in the foundation of the Diabetic Association of Australia, later the Diabetic Association of New South Wales.) He described the dreadful situation faced by Type 1 diabetics before 1922 and also the miraculous arrival of insulin:

> I recall opening the door of a certain male medical ward and being assailed by the strong and sickly-sweet smell of acetone. Most of the patients were lying down singly, weak, thin, thirsty and disinterested. The bedside notes recorded progressive weight loss, constant heavy glycosuria [sugar in the urine] and frequent urinary ketosis [acidic breakdown of fats in the urine]. Their low carbohydrate diet included twice boiled green vegetables, virtually no bread or starchy food, a modest serving of meat or fish, restricted fruit and salt. The importance of high vitamin foods, and still less of commercially prepared tablets, was not yet realised. The importance of calcium was also unrecognised at this time. Fat was unrestricted, including cream. Furuncles [boils], minor abrasions and skin traumas healed slowly or not at all, particularly in the lower extremities. Attempts at cutting corns and nails and ill-fitting footwear could be the starting point of gangrene which could spread inexorably up the limb until high level amputation became inevitable.
>
> Within a year, crude insulin, in small quantities obtained from [animal pancreas via] the slaughterhouse, became available, and with unforgettable excitement we saw miraculous changes. The slightly cloudy insulin was not yet standardised, and doses were largely experimental. Localised reactions were universal,

but worthwhile as both physician and patient shared the same thrilling experience of using the new animal hormone.

Dr Elliot Joslin, a famous American authority, wrote: 'I am reminded of the words of the prophet Ezekiel. No better description of the transformation in the life of the advanced diabetic exists than the prophet's vision of the "valley of dry bones" (Ezekiel XXXVII 5–10, King James Version):

> *Thus saith the Lord God to these bones: Behold I will cause breath to enter into you and ye shall live. And I will lay sinews upon you and will bring up flesh to grow upon you, and cover you with skin . . . And when I beheld, lo, the sinews and the flesh came up upon them, and the skin covered them . . . and the breath came into them and they lived, and they stood up upon their feet, an exceeding great army.'*

This immediate transformation, within a few days of insulin administration, was one of the most memorable I have ever seen, and never forgotten by the physicians and students of my generation.

Sir John Kempson Maddox died in Sydney on 27 July 1990.

Early insulin was quick acting, so that many injections were needed through the day—and the ability to monitor the level of glucose in the blood was not developed until the late 1930s and 1940s. Soon longer acting insulin was developed, using protamine (extracted from fish testes), zinc and insulin.

After the 1960s insulin was purified to a greater extent than before because of better techniques, but it was still coming from pigs (whose insulin is only one amino acid different from humans) and beef cattle (two amino acids different). There were rare allergic reactions to this animal-derived insulin, and some disfigurement at injection sites.

The next big breakthrough came in the 1980s with the development in the United States of genetically engineered insulin, which replaced animal insulin (which is still available in some countries and, for special circumstances, in Australia).

At the beginning of the twenty-first century, children with Type 1 diabetes quickly learn to inject themselves with a choice of specially developed insulin pens—or syringes—which use fine needles and which are almost completely painless. Indeed, users say that the injection routine hurts less than routine finger pricking to test BGL (blood glucose levels). There are now special automatic pumps which can deliver the correct amount of insulin throughout the day. These are small devices worn around the waist, under clothing, which feed the insulin through a small catheter, enabling young people to go to school, play sport, work and socialise with their peers unshackled from their daily injection routine and allow immediate adjustment of insulin to suit meals and activities.

Up until the discovery and extraction of insulin in 1922 the only outcome for Type 1 diabetes was an illness that was inevitably fatal. Even up to and just after World War II, treatment was an inexact science. Children of that era who survive to this day tell Dickensian stories of battling diabetes.

Bruce Beal

Evacuated to England from Burma as a small child before World War II, Bruce Beal began his life in England by being taken into care and reared in a workhouse (Dickens would have been proud) before he was boarded out with his maternal grandmother, whom he had never met before then. During the war he and his grandmother were bombed out of their house twice. The family next door—including his playmates—were all killed.

Bruce's fortunes lifted briefly when he won a scholarship to train as a choir boy at an English cathedral. He loved both the school attached and the singing, and a high point was being picked—two years running—as the soloist to sing the opening carol at the Christmas service. He hoped for a trifecta, but his voice broke and that was the end of both the choir and the school. With no home to go back to, he was taken to live at a medieval priory in West Sussex. He also developed diabetes, but his loss of weight, severe headaches and swollen ankles were all put down to stress and unhappiness at leaving the choir school.

Just before Christmas 1947 he was admitted to the children's hospital at Brighton. It was not a good time to be seriously ill. The National Health Service had not yet been set up in Britain, and the best hospitals had been requisitioned by the government for injured servicemen. There were no antibiotics available and poliomyelitis and diphtheria carried off children in droves. Staff were largely untrained as the best nurses were still attached to the military hospitals. Bruce and other seriously ill children were cared for by poorly paid, ill-educated sixteen-year-old girls.

Bathing was unheard of. Washing was performed at the bed using chamber pots. There was no flush toilet in the ward, and only one bath and wash basin for patients. The hospitals were breeding grounds for infection, not helped by the sanitary standards. The bed legs stood in metal saucers filled with Jeyes Fluid, a disinfectant, in the hope that fleas and lice would drown while making the crossing. 'Sadly,' Bruce said, 'the little varmints developed great skill in leaping over these obstacles'.

As a teenager he was diagnosed with nephritis (inflammation of the kidneys) and diabetes. The only insulin available in the

UK came from the cattle industry and was impure, Bruce recalled, and very difficult to take:

> The needles were huge and we would have to cut them to a size to suit us and then sharpen them on a special stone. The glass syringe for injection was kept in a glass dish filled with alcohol, which would remain in the dish until the alcohol had gone black. At that time we only had a short-term insulin of very uncertain purity. The injection was once a day and was terribly painful. We would spend ages trying to sharpen our needle on the stone to try and make the injection more comfortable. We know now that all our efforts were a waste of time. We would simply make the point even more jagged and more likely to tear the flesh and cause a severe infection.
>
> Later we had Marshall Plan Lilly insulin and moved to two injections per day. It was in short supply and we used the minimum doses to maintain life. Home glucose testing did not start for me until 1968 and blood glucose testing started for me on 12 November 1979.

Tom Beatson

Tom Beatson was diagnosed in 1942, one month after his tenth birthday following his collapse into a coma. His family was then living in New Rochelle, a suburb of New York City. He had long periods of hospitalisation to try and stabilise his condition—fortunately under better circumstances than Bruce Beale in the United Kingdom.

As soon as he was able to, Tom was taught to test his blood sugar, and inject insulin. The testing was quite elaborate:

> For the first couple of years I had to rely on urine tests with Benedict's solution. Benedict's solution was a fancy name for copper sulfate solution. We bought it in quart-sized (or larger) bottles at the local pharmacy, measured a couple of inches of it into a test tube, added a specified number of drops of urine, put the test tube into a metal measuring cup with a couple of inches of water, and boiled it for about five minutes on the gas stove in the kitchen. The natural solution was dark blue but if there was sugar in the urine the heat caused the color to change to bright orange.
>
> There was a color chart for determining whether the result was 'negative', or 1+, 2+, 3+, or 4+. After the war was over, one company started making copper sulfate tablets, and timed burning tablets. They packaged them in a case and included a test tube and a clamp to hold the test tube.

Injecting insulin was no less elaborate. As in the United Kingdom, insulin was a by-product of the slaughter of beef cattle. Tom's father bought it in quantity, five 10cc vials at a time. (Interestingly enough, diabetic measurements were always in the metric system in the United States even though they have still not changed over from the imperial system.) There were also different glass-barrelled syringes for different strengths of insulin. During puberty, Tom said, he was injecting himself with more than 80 units of insulin in one shot—a huge dose:

> My mother was taught to inject, but she only injected me when it was necessary to use my arms (because I couldn't pinch my own arm and inject myself). While on one injection a day I always used the thighs, even though the doses were large, and my thighs got kind of lumpy.

Insulin time line

1921	Insulin discovered by Dr Banting and Dr Best.
1922	Leonard Thompson, a 14-year-old, became the first human to receive insulin extracts from Dr Collip.
1922	Eli Lilly and Company and the University of Toronto formed a partnership to produce insulin in bulk.
1923	Dr Banting and Professor Macleod awarded the Nobel Prize in Physiology or Medicine for their research into diabetes.
1940s	Scientists discovered a connection between diabetes and kidney and eye diseases.
1944	Standard insulin syringe is prepared.
1950s	Research of DNA to make a form of human insulin began.
1955	New drugs to be taken orally developed to help lower the blood glucose level.
1959	Scientists categorised diabetes into two forms: Type 1 for those dependent on insulin, and Type 2 non-insulin dependent.
1970	Blood glucose meters and insulin pumps developed.
1983	First biosynthetic human insulin introduced.
1986	Insulin pen delivery system developed.
1996	The Food and Drug Administration in the United States approves human insulin made from DNA.
1996	Throughout the world the 75th anniversary of the discovery of insulin celebrated.

Peter Corris

The Australian author and crime writer, Peter Corris, had unwieldy injection and testing procedures to cope with when he became ill with Type 1 diabetes in 1958 at the age of sixteen. Writing about his diabetic experiences in a candid memoir, *Sweet & Sour—A Diabetic Life*, Peter remarked that people diagnosed with diabetes in the past twenty years would find the technology used in the 1950s and 1960s like something out of the stone age:

> Instead of light, disposable plastic syringes, sealed swabs and pen injectors, we stored our glass and metal syringes and three needles (one for drawing up the insulin, one for injecting and a spare) in screw-top plastic containers filled with surgical spirit. Swabbing was done with cotton wool and methylated spirits—a bottle to be kept filled . . . but the spirit became milky after a time and had to be changed. The needles had to be sterilised each week by boiling, a tiresome task for a teenager.

Testing for blood sugar would be revolutionised in the 1970s with the development of the computerised glucometer, enabling BGL to be monitored by pricking the side of a finger and getting a result in a matter of seconds. This enabled both doctors and diabetics to achieve good control. In 1958, when Peter faced up to his diabetes, the only method was to test urine for the presence of sugar. It was messy, complicated and, worse, not very accurate. To test, it was necessary to piddle into a plastic cup and then use a supplied kit, which held a test tube, eye dropper and 'reagent' tablets:

> The kit came with a chart for recording the results of each test. The chart was submitted to the endocrinologist periodically for review of one's 'control', a fiddly, boring procedure. I am sure I was not the only young diabetic to lie about it—to tell my parents I had tested when I had not, to neglect to enter the results or to falsify them. Still worse, urine testing did not really work.

While he was first waiting to be diagnosed, the teenage Peter read an article about diabetes in *Readers' Digest* in the doctor's waiting room. It had some positive things to say—mentioning that the great American tennis players Bill Talbert and Ham Richardson had diabetes—but went on to detail the downside of the disease, an increased risk of heart disease, a high incidence of blindness and in males ('the word struck a fear into my heart that remained with me for almost forty years') . . . *impotence*!

Corris said he later learned that vascular damage of all kinds was thought to be an inevitable consequence of diabetes, however supposedly good the 'control':

> Despite the much publicised athletic successes of Talbert and Richardson and the intellectual achievements of such diabetics as H. G. Wells, there was a public perception of the diabetic as a frail, flawed creature. This was brought home sharply to me early in the '60s in the film *Hud*. In one scene Paul Newman is trying to placate the husband he has just cuckolded: 'Now Joe, you know you've got sugar diabetes.'

No fun to be cast as the cuckold rather than the stud.

Shortly after adjusting to his new diabetic routine, Peter had his first hypo (hypoglycaemic) attack, a drastic fall in the blood sugar level causing heavy sweating, mental weakness and mental confusion. It was during his school holidays, and in this case was due to over-exertion at some activity, lawn mowing or sport, without taking some sugar to retain the balance:

> I sat in a chair in the living room on a warm afternoon and felt very peculiar. I had never sweated like this before; it was soaking my clothes and dripping into my eyes. My vision was affected by that and something else . . . a kind of distancing tunnel vision that made close objects seem small and far away. My mother found me before the level dropped too low and mixed a sickly sugar and milk drink that brought me out of it. I have had many such episodes since, and my saviour has always been a woman.

As Peter Corris makes clear in his book, he has not let diabetes dominate his life, in the course of which he has had three professions—academic, journalist and writer—travelled to many countries and lived in all three of the eastern Australian states. He has been married twice and became a parent to three children. One of the reasons he wrote about his diabetes was to help some people avoid the mistakes he made. At the time of writing, Peter had had diabetes for 41 years. For the first 20 of those he was angry and in denial, as he wrote, 'setting myself on a course that would have led to blindness, amputation and an early death'. For the past 21 years he has been behaving as a diabetic should, 'a long downward swoop and an upturn just in time'.

His change in attitude came in 1978 when he was 36 years old, through a meeting with the outspoken medico, Professor Fred Hollows, after having laser treatment for diabetic retinopathy, which saved his sight. The full account can be read in Peter Corris's book, but this is the moment that turned him around:

> [Hollows] looked at me over the tops of his half-glasses, took the curved pipe out of his mouth, and prodded me hard in my soft belly with his fist.
>
> 'What's this gut you've got on you? You've had all this expensive treatment and you're just fucking throwing it away. Diabetics should be thin! If you don't get off the piss and get fit you'll be blind in five years and dead in ten.'

When I read this I was reminded of Doctor Ron's fairly forthright comment to me about the possibility of blindness and amputation when I asked what would happen if I ignored my late onset Type 2 diabetes. While not facing the challenges that Peter Corris, as a Type 1 diabetic, had to face as a young man, I could still suffer the same side effects if I was dopey enough to ignore an incurable disease. Since my diagnosis I have spoken to many people with Type 2 diabetes who were not spoken to as bluntly or directly by the GPs as I had been, and as a result seemed unaware of the dangers to their health that awaited them.

Geoff, a retired university senior lecturer, who developed Type 2 diabetes at age 60, thinks he remained undiagnosed for at least four years, even after doing an executive stress test and having a thorough medical going over. The GP who looked at his results commented that he had a BGL higher than the therapeutic range (which is from 4 to 8 mmol/L) and might be diabetic, but did not suggest that he have further tests, or say anything about diabetes and its dangers. Geoff didn't know what a BGL was anyway, like most people to this day!

> I didn't know what diabetes was. I had no symptoms and how could I have a chronic, potentially deadly illness when I'm still going down to the gym three to four times a week and

> swimming 80 laps in the pool? When I'm still putting in 12-hour days at the university giving lectures to 500 students without notes? So how could I be sick?

Four years later, after having felt desperately ill for a week, Geoff collapsed at his home, fortunately managing to phone his ex-wife although he was barely conscious. When he arrived at the hospital, collapsing again in the foyer, his BGL was 26.5 mmol/L—high enough to result in a hyperglycaemic coma—and he required immediate treatment.

The onset of Type 2 diabetes, although not as dramatic as Type 1 with the total loss of insulin production by the pancreas, is nonetheless extremely serious. I am one of the lucky ones, as I discovered, able to control it by diet and exercise—for the moment. Geoff is not so lucky, and his life and retirement years have already been plagued by chronic illness, mostly related to his diabetes. (I'll talk more about his unfortunate situation in the next chapter.)

By 1959, research scientists differentiated Type 1 and Type 2 diabetes. Before then, they had been lumped together. Rosalyn Yalow and Sol Berson 'invented' radioimmunoassay—which included a way to detect very small amounts of hormones in blood—and were able to measure insulin levels in blood for the first time. They worked out that Type 2 diabetes was a condition with *high* insulin levels (an insulin resistant state), and Type 1 was diabetes with *no* insulin (an insulin deficient state). The science of radioimmunoassay testing developed by Yalow and Berson in New York led to modern endocrinology as we know it today. Yalow won the Nobel Prize for Medicine in 1977 for her work—only the second woman to win a Nobel in the history of the prize.

The main difference between the two diabetic conditions is that unlike people with Type 1, those with Type 2 diabetes are still producing insulin, but their bodies are not processing it properly. Unfortunately there are no immediate or obvious symptoms and people—like Geoff—can go undiagnosed for years before collapsing with sky-high glucose levels in their blood, or until diabetic symptoms such as excessive unquenchable thirst, urinating too much, or having trouble with their eyes become apparent.

Those with type 2 diabetes (NIDDM) can suffer the same dire side effects as Type 1 (IDDM), either unknowingly, or by going into denial about their diabetic status. Paradoxically, although Type 2 diabetes is called 'non-insulin dependent diabetes', some patients do progress to the need for daily insulin injections to manage their disease. This is why, in the 1990s, the term NIDDM was changed to Type 2 diabetes and IDDM, or insulin dependent diabetes, was changed to Type 1 diabetes.

As I've said before it's been estimated that 90 per cent of people with diabetes have Type 2—that is 1.2 million Australians. But only half of these actually know that they have it! Type 2 diabetes is Australia's fastest growing chronic disease. By the year 2010, Diabetes Australia expects there will be 1.8 million people with Type 2—and it isn't only old farts like me who are getting it. There is a disturbing rise in the incidence of insulin resistance (a precursor to Type 2 diabetes) and Type 2 cases in quite young children and in those in early adolescence. Researchers are still trying to find out why. Is it a combination of too much junk food, lack of exercise and vegging out in front of the telly or computer games, or some other environmental or even a genetic reason? The answer is probably a combination of genes and the environment—too little physical activity and too much food, especially junk food.

The costs to the health service and the country are massive. There is still no cure for either Type 1 or Type 2 diabetes. Medical researchers hope they will discover a cure for Type 1 diabetes fairly soon. No one is saying that, however, about Type 2, which for the moment has to be managed. However, a number of recent studies have shown that the onset of Type 2 diabetes can be prevented or at least delayed by lifestyle strategies as simple as healthy eating habits and regular exercise. On that front, the news gets more positive, as further research into diabetic management yields better and better results—not only with diet and exercise, but superior drugs as well.

CHAPTER FOUR

I don't have any symptoms

I actually said it myself when I was diagnosed with Type 2 diabetes: 'But I don't have any symptoms!' That is the insidious part of diabetes. You can have it for years, sometimes, and not know until there is some kind of medical event—problems with eyesight, perhaps the sensation of burning feet or infections that won't heal—before a diagnosis is made. Such events mean real damage may have been done, which could have been avoided with early detection. I probably only just slipped over the bar from glucose intolerance—a pre-diabetic condition from which you may pull back from full-blown Type 2 diabetes mellitus—about a year before diagnosis. I have since learned that one third of people who have pre-diabetes progress to Type 2 diabetes, one third remain with pre-diabetes and one third revert to normal. The good news is that recent studies have shown that with simple alterations to lifestyle, such as exercise and healthy eating, diabetes may be delayed or prevented in about 58 per cent of people with pre-diabetes.

Had I known where I was heading, perhaps I would have done something about it. I say 'perhaps', because there is a raft of difference between 'having' a disease and 'might get it'. That's the real challenge of preventive medicine. Getting people to think ahead. Obesity in the United States, and Australia, is putting enormous (adjectives in this area tend towards bursting semantic seams) strains on national health systems as fatties develop heart disease and a raft of other predictable medical problems because their overloaded bodies pack it in under the strain of it all. And that is one gigantic (there I go again) reason why more and more of us are developing diabetes.

So I'm not sure whether I would have been 'Mr Goody Two-Shoes' if I had been alerted at the pre-diabetic glucose intolerance stage. It's a bit like a soldier in battle: The bullets are for the others, not for me. Of course I know better now . . .

I had some awareness of the importance of having my blood pressure and cholesterol monitored, but the idea of blood sugar testing (the BGL) had never occurred to me. When I was picked up on a routine health check on reaching the ripe age of 65, I asked my GP, Ron, who practises in retirement heartland, if he ordered BGL tests on all his patients:

Ron: Well anyone over a certain age or with certain risk factors. I think anyone over 55 who's never been tested and those over 45 with another risk factor, such as high blood pressure, even if they don't have a family history, should have a BGL test. Most people over 55 should know what their cholesterol level is, their triglycerides [forms of fat] are, their sugar level, of course, and in males especially, their liver function. Most people in Australia tend to drink moderately or more than moderately so liver's often done as well. And you also find that fatty liver is more common in people with diabetes as well as high cholesterol and other things.

Tim: I told you I couldn't possibly have diabetes. Is that a fairly typical reaction?

Ron: Ah yes, people don't believe it because people remember what diabetics were like 20 or 30 years ago, which means they remember people with their legs cut off—my grandmother died a horrible death with gangrene. I haven't actually seen a gangrenous leg for at least ten years, which means the management has improved immeasurably in that time—as has vascular surgery and other things. That's why people are so shocked, because mild diabetes is almost a normal age-related thing. If everyone lived to 90, there's going to be a high proportion of people who have at least impaired glucose tolerance, if not diabetes.

Tim: But I've talked to people who have been diagnosed late in life and they said their GP was a bit casual about it: 'It's a by-product of lifestyle, you must expect it', sort of thing. One man of my vintage finished up in a coma with blood levels of 25 [mmol/L] and even higher!

Ron: A lot depends on the GP. I've had plenty of patients who have moved from the city, where they had been told, 'You've got a bit of sugar, but don't worry'. And their sugars are 14 and 15 and we all know at that level they may corrode their arteries and go blind or suffer kidney problems. So it's not like the 1940s or 50s any more when people used to say, 'Oh you've got a bit of sugar'. The main reason they used to say that was because they couldn't do anything about it in those days. But that's not the right attitude now.

Because of where I live, with a large retirement population, I was lucky to find Ron, who is constantly on the alert for diabetes. He estimated that at least 20 per cent of his patients had diabetes, with a further 10 per cent in the pre-diabetes phrase of glucose intolerance (that is a fasting BGL of between 6.1 and 6.9 mmol/L, or tests two hours after a meal between 7.8 and 11 mmol/L).

Not everyone gets such good initial care. I spoke to Paul, a 40-year-old journalist who was diagnosed about the same time I was. He was living in Queensland at the time:

Paul: I was staying with my parents in Toowoomba after returning from working in Hong Kong. I was fairly inactive during a prolonged 'holiday', doing not much more than vegging out on the couch and playing the occasional game of golf. Every now and then I started to feel a bit nauseous, which persisted for a day or two. I was also dropping off to sleep after my evening meals (that's despite an espresso coffee I almost always have). One day after a walk into the town centre and an afternoon trying to kill time (which is harder than it sounds in Toowoomba) I was shaky and sweaty when I returned home. My mum thought I'd been propping up a bar somewhere, but I hadn't had a drop. I was very agitated and hungry and *had* to eat immediately. A quick surf on the Internet and a visit to the doctor the next day confirmed my earlier suspicions—I had diabetes.

Tim: How did your doctor break the news to you?

Paul: Quite brutally. Before he took my BGL I had told him, after my amateur diagnosis on the net, that I suspected I had diabetes. After recording a whopping 17 mmol/L on the blood prick test his exact words were, 'Congratulations, you have diabetes'. He didn't hold his punches. He told me my days as a 'hard-living, hard-drinking' journalist were over, adding that if I chose to ignore my condition it would, 'Get me, and get me in a horrible way'. When I offered the feeble, 'Why me, I'm still young plea', he answered, 'What do you expect, you're 40, overweight and inactive'. Ouch! Harsh words, but so far they've done the trick.

Tim: How did you react to the diagnosis at first?

Paul: A bit nonplussed. A sense of doom that the sweet life had been brought to a shattering end, but also a sense of relief knowing what was wrong with me and what I had to do if I wanted to live a long, healthy life. I'd been drafted into the Diabetes Corp for the remainder of my life and there was no shore leave.

Paul took his diabetes seriously, joined Diabetes Australia in Brisbane, sought the advice of a dietitian (although he did not go to any group sessions), modified his diet and began an exercise program to lose weight. This was important, because at 5 foot 8 inches [1.72 metres] he was just over 100 kilograms. He immediately began his exercise program of mainly walking and climbing stairs instead of taking the lift. He said he began testing his blood sugars rather obsessively at first, up to four times a day, and was surprised to find—within a week—that he was within the normal range. However, like me, he still had diabetes. As a fellow journalist, I asked him about grog:

Paul: Oh yes, the alcohol question. I was quite a heavy drinker before the epiphany. In fact pain under my rib cage, both sides, was what started the alarm bells ringing in terms of general concerns over my health. I suspected my liver wasn't the greatest, but even my rudimentary understanding of

> human anatomy had me puzzling about pain on the left side. My liver couldn't be there—unless it had grown to the size of a ham hock and was annexing the rest of my torso for future invasions. When I was diagnosed with diabetes they also tested my kidneys and liver. Indeed, my liver wasn't the greatest but the new lifestyle has gone some way towards repairing the damage (and I'd invested so much time and money defiling my own temple). But I'm no saint. I usually have two to three schooners of light beer a day or a few glasses of red wine. Alcohol-free days are a struggle, particularly when surrounded by Olympic-class tipplers. As a footnote, I found a brief period of total abstinence counter-productive on the 'Enjoyment-Of-Life-I'm-Turning-Into-A-Total-Dweb' index.

A feeling I well understand and I am a quarter-of-a-century older than Paul.

Only a matter of weeks after he was diagnosed, Paul moved to Sydney to work as a sub-editor on a daily newspaper. He needed another doctor, but wasn't too impressed by his first experience. When Paul said he would need more information, the medico said that he could email him, and he would respond at a charge of $50 per question! 'Maybe', said Paul, 'it's a Sydney thing. Perhaps he's wearing fishnet stockings and gold-hooped earrings when he types'.

I wondered where this email suggestion registered on the scale of medical ethics. Paul, when I last spoke to him, was on the trail of more diabetes-friendly medical advice and referral to a diabetes centre for education after contacting Diabetes Australia–NSW. It is not my aim to indulge in doctor bashing, but there is a good deal of anecdotal evidence to suggest a number of medicos are not as aware of diabetes as they might be, nor do some of them take it seriously enough. This is probably more so, as my country-based GP Ron suggested earlier, in city practices where GPs treat a patient who presents once with a particular problem and who might not return to that practice.

An unfortunate combination of late diagnosis, and the onset of Type 2 diabetes, was the situation faced by Geoff, the university academic I mentioned briefly in the previous chapter. We met by chance at the Sydney Writers' Festival in 2003, following the talks I gave on my diabetes diagnosis on the ABC's Radio National's *Health Report*. Geoff had heard the talks and made himself known to me. I found his story extraordinary, and we met later to talk about it. If anyone had lucked out on Type 2 diabetes, it was Geoff.

Several years before Geoff elected to retire from his university, he was sent to a hot-shot diagnostic centre for executives—one of those places where you flash your credit card and undergo a battery of tests ranging from blood analysis to one of those treadmills where your heart is monitored while you run yourself ragged. I did one of these in the 1980s when you could do it on Medicare with no extra charges. In fact Medicare probably sustained these glittering palaces of prognostication.

(I recall the ABC's then newly appointed Director of Television, Richard Thomas, did one of these executive medical makeovers in the early 1980s. As I understand it, he actually had a heart attack on the treadmill, monitored by a doctor, who watched it happen on his screen. Instead of calling an ambulance, he told Richard that he had some heart problems and should seek further medical advice! After swiping his corporate card they couldn't get him off the premises quickly enough. Some hours after he got home—which is often the case—he suffered another, but more major, coronary and very nearly died.)

Geoff was a very fit man in his late fifties when he did one of these diagnostic makeovers in 1997. At least the doctor who oversaw his results said: 'Go and see your doctor. You might be diabetic.' Geoff didn't know anything about diabetes, but dutifully did as he was told. His GP told him his all-over results were terrific. 'But what about diabetes?' His doctor looked at the therapeutic range and said he thought it looked okay to him. Unfortunately Geoff can't remember what the BGL figures were, because they didn't mean anything to him at that stage.

He decided to retire at the end of 1999, and put in his letter of resignation to the university in June—feeling rather excited and pleased with this decision and full of plans for an active retirement. Three weeks later he started feeling most unwell, and thought he had the 'flu. He went to his GP, who was away, and saw a colleague on duty at the time. He said it seemed as though Geoff had the 'flu and that he should take it easy for a week. Geoff said it seemed a funny sort of 'flu, because he was forever peeing and was having to drink at least three litres of liquid during the night. He asked the doctor why he needed to drink so much? Now excessive urination and thirst are classic symptoms of diabetes, but it rang no bells with this doctor. 'He didn't respond to this, but just told me to go home and lie down because there wasn't anything really that could be done about 'flu.'

Geoff, who lives alone, did what he was told, and took the week off. But a week later, on a Saturday, he still felt absolutely dreadful:

Tim: So what happened?

Geoff: I got out of bed and I thought I've got to go to hospital—I had never been taken to hospital through illness in my whole life! I got as far as the middle of the living room, and stood immobile. I couldn't move. I thought, 'This isn't the 'flu'. I had enough brain cells left to get to the phone and ring my ex-wife, Margo, with whom I have an excellent relationship. Fortunately she only lives one suburb away. I said, 'Get over here quickly—I literally think I'm dying'. She's known me for 43 years, and was aware I was in good shape. She came in her car, took me down to my GP—my real GP this time—and he wrote out a referral letter to the hospital for admission. We went to my local public hospital because it was nearest, only to be informed that there were no beds. Margo said, 'Take one look at him—by the time I get him to the next hospital he's going to be dead!' A nurse came and took my BGL and it was 26.6 mmol/L. Margo made things happen, God bless her.

So they put me on a trolley and parked me somewhere. This would have been about 10.30 a.m. At about 4 p.m., having seen a younger doctor earlier in the morning, a very senior doctor came along to see me and I was shaking and rattling and rolling and almost out of it. He admitted me to hospital and I was in there for five days.

Tim: Were you conscious during that time?

Geoff: Well the first day only more or less. If someone had said, 'Fire, everybody out', I'm afraid I couldn't have responded to that. So five days. They put me on insulin and I had some diabetes education. I was told how to administer the insulin by the hospital diabetes educator. When I came out I decided that I had been so badly treated by my GP over the last three or so years, I needed to change my doctor.

Tim: Who had failed to recognise classic symptoms of diabetes . . .

Geoff: Absolutely. I didn't know what diabetes was at the time. I'd never had any abrasions with the medical profession of a serious nature. I was ruggedly healthy. So I came back and went to another GP, explaining the circumstances. He said, 'Well you've got to test your blood sugar levels every day and the best way to do that is to pee onto these testing strips.'

Tim: You're kidding!

Geoff: I wish I was. He said, 'You pee on these strips and if it comes up this colour your blood glucose level is right, and it should be between 4 and 8. Pee on these strips once or twice a day, and record the results in a little book. So I went along to the pharmacist with an order for these strips and the pharmacist was surprised to say the least. I said, 'I need these strips to pee on'. He said, 'Really? I'm not sure we've got any. I don't think I've seen any around here for 20 years'. I said, 'Oh, well it must be an obscure disease then if this is what I have to do'. Of course I now know glucometers to check blood glucose levels have been around since the 1970s.

Tim: That doctor is probably still prescribing laudanum [tincture of opium].

Geoff: After a couple of weeks I began to realise he was a bit of a dill. He was way past retirement age, and probably hadn't read, or even glanced at the medical journals in 20 years. I went to another GP who had been recommended to me by a friend of mine who was also a diabetic.

I went to this guy and I told him my sad story and he immediately had all my records faxed from the hospital into his office—they were there within ten minutes. He got me onto the table, examined me, gave me a reference to go to a diabetes expert who gave me a 90-minute examination. He sent me off to a heart specialist to have my heart checked, an eye doctor to have my eyes checked, and a podiatrist to check my feet for neuropathy. He also said, 'Go to the dentist and get your teeth checked. I'll give you a certificate for six weeks off work because you're going to be a very busy boy seeing all these people'. This was several weeks after discharge from hospital and my readings were still 16.6 mmol/L. This is still a very high blood sugar level.

Tim: You're injecting insulin in the meantime are you?

Geoff: I was for a while, but my new doctor had taken me off insulin and put me on medication. He said, 'We'll try it without insulin—I don't want you to be on insulin if we can avoid it'.

Tim: Of course, it was believed that you were Type 2 by now.

Geoff: Yes. The doctor said, 'Has anybody told you about Diabetes Australia and the NDSS scheme?' I said no. He said, 'Has anybody told you about diabetes education?' I said no. I had been to my previous GP, by the way, some three or four months before this, saying that I seem to be drinking a lot and peeing a lot—but no lights came on, no lights at all. And he said, 'Why haven't you been informed?' I said, 'Look, it's not my policy to badmouth people with whom I've had professional dealings because you're only hearing one side of the story'. He told me to get myself up to the diabetes centre quick smart and enrol in diabetes education classes, which I did. I was still so unwell that I ended up having the entire six months of my pre-retirement period off work, in fact I never worked again. I was off work for six months and I was still so sick come my retirement date of December 31 that my retirement luncheon was deferred until February 28 because I was still too ill to go to the university.

Geoff is still in a bad way. Before he was stricken with diabetes, his health was excellent. He had a couple of orthopaedic procedures on his knees, but that was about it. He told me he looked forward to fronting up to retirement, vigorous and strong. But he spent the next two years, after collapsing with stratospheric blood sugar levels, feeling like 'a sick man'. 'I suddenly felt older and more frail. I was no longer able to go down to the pool and do 80 laps—I was a good swimmer. I wasn't able to do good gym workouts and all that stuff, and I found going out at night difficult.'

After a particularly virulent urinary tract infection—bacterial prostatitis—he relapsed six months later with another bout, and had half his prostate removed. 'As a result of that I'm now basically out of the sexual game—that doesn't bother me—as there was cancer in that area.'

Tim: Was that operation in any way associated with your diabetes?

Geoff: People develop prostate problems for reasons other than being diabetic, but being diabetic enhances the possibility that you may develop an infection in that area . . .

Tim: Certainly it's known that diabetes can cause erectile dysfunction.

Geoff: I have erectile dysfunction. Absolutely. I was actually told by my GP to go out and buy a *Playboy* and see if it did anything for me! So I went into a newsagency, not in my suburb, and I can assure you it did nothing for me at all. The girls looked wonderful, but they had no impact. I thought, 'Geoff, what's life come to?' Now I have another problem. I ended up in hospital in distressing circumstances in February 2002 with all the classic symptoms of left-lobe temporal epilepsy. They had me wired up to all manner of high-tech equipment and while I was monitored by the intensive care unit I had a major drama which saw doctors (including my new neurologist who just happened to be in the ward) scurrying to my side. Margo was there and saw it all. I had no awareness of what was going on.

Tim: You had fits?

Geoff: Yes. I've been on medication for that ever since and I see my neurologist every six months, and I have regular MRI [Magnetic Resonance Imaging] scans.

Tim: Has the medication controlled it?

Geoff: By and large. In August this year my medication was increased by 25 per cent. In the last six months I've only had two major attacks, which is a lot better than the two to three attacks per week I was having. This, like diabetes, is a progressively degenerative disease which medication can control but not cure.

Tim: What happens when you have one of these attacks?

Geoff: A left-lobe temporal epilepsy fit is quite curious. You can be proceeding about your daily life and then suddenly you stop, and you stare, and the world around you seems to compress and rushes in and stops about three to four feet away. I just stand there sweating violently, sometimes talking to myself. If somebody shouts, 'Get off the road you silly bugger or the bus will knock you over', I will have no understanding of that. Within two to three minutes it clears up. Then I can get on with what I am doing, continue walking if I am out, or start vacuuming the floor again, or playing the piano.

Tim: Do you have to sit down or can you stand up?

Geoff: You just freeze in either position. I had a classic one outside the Art Gallery one day in the rain when I was with Margo. I stopped, holding an umbrella above my head, shielding both of us for three minutes, while I had one of these attacks.

Tim: Did she know?

Geoff: Yes, she's seen it heaps of times and knows not to interfere. I didn't drop the umbrella. Everything stopped. It was a cold, wet day and I was sweating like a pig. Then it stopped within three minutes and we proceeded into the Art Gallery to hear a one-hour lecture. Then we had lunch and everything was just normal. Recently I had one in a bus and alarmed people nearby who thought I was having a heart attack. I have had many such public attacks.

Geoff believes that both these medical conditions may be related to his diabetes, but it can't be proved. Two GPs and both his specialists have 'vaguely' suggested such a connection. On top of everything else, the stabilisation of his diabetes is proving to be extremely difficult. His present doctor is juggling his medication to try and bring his blood glucose levels down rather than progress to insulin. His blood levels can be in the normal range of 4 to 5 mmol/L one day, and soar to 11 or 13 or down to 3 the next. Unfortunately his knees are also playing up and he can't exercise as much as he needs to. The only alternative is a major knee reconstruction, which he is waiting to have done. But there is an added concern about undergoing prolonged anaesthesia. With his recent track record of emerging damaged from operations, Geoff is apprehensive about the procedure but plans to go ahead nevertheless. He has brought his weight down from 92 to 76 kilos.

As if to prove the axiom that there is no justice in matters of health, there are also concerns about his kidney function. A recent haemorrhoidectomy did not go well, leaving a legacy of violent spasms of pain that were bad enough to put him back in hospital for four days, just before Geoff and I met to discuss his case. It is not surprising to learn that he was extremely depressed about his situation and his future:

Tim: How are you faring psychologically?

Geoff: Damaged. You get out of bed of a morning, wander around, and you do your blood glucose reading, have breakfast, make your bed, wash up and play a bit of piano and you do your two-hour BGL after a meal, only to find you're 12.7 mmol/L. You know the way to get that down is to go for a 40-minute walk but you can't because your knee-caps are clapped out, you begin to think, 'I'm one of the good guys, this shouldn't be happening'. Had I been properly diagnosed and treated back in September 1997, maybe a lot of this would not have happened. I'm not the sort of person who creates sensations and makes waves so the prospect of bringing lawsuits and alleging this and badmouthing people etc. is not my style. It's happened, it's happened.

I'm a victim, I feel I'm a victim. It could have been handled better but I've never badmouthed the three GPs who mismanaged my situation from 1997 to June 1999—I never have and never will. I've certainly spoken about this to Margo of course, but I've fallen on better times in the sense that I'm now properly managed by a range of experts whom I see regularly. I feel my situation is being properly managed even though I do seem to be constantly popping into hospital for this and that. When we were coming back from hospital last Thursday I said to Margo, 'Thank God that's over. With any sort of luck, if the knee caps hold out, I might go another year without having to go into hospital'. I was back in hospital that night. Woke up in one hospital and went to bed in another that same night.

Tim: Even though there's no justice in matters of health, I think you could do with a bit of good news?

Geoff: I would welcome some good news—but it's not going to get good. Diabetes takes over your life in a way that no other disease does. If you're going to have, say, a knee reconstruction, you're diagnosed, you go to hospital, you spend two weeks in hospital, you're on crutches for eight weeks, you're on a walking stick for six months and then you're cured. But with diabetes, it is an unending life commitment dealing not only with your readings, your daily illnesses but all the other dysfunctional consequences that arise. I don't think I would be able to handle my diabetes and hold down the position I held at my old university. I would be taking so much time off work that I think I would become an absolute nuisance for somebody, even at my senior level.

Tim: But you also, it would have to be said, drew the short straw on being an atypical case of Type 2 diabetes?

Geoff: Indeed, but I think there are a sufficient number of atypical cases. I met a number of them when I was in hospital about a year ago. There were three men my age in a single room. I said to the nurse one day, 'Why have you got us four buggers in the one room, when there are empty beds up and down the ward. Why can't you give us a bit of space?'

She said, 'You're all over 60, you're all male, you're all diabetic, you're all seriously ill and you're right opposite the nurses station'.

The guy opposite me had had one leg amputated thanks to neuropathy. The man next to me used to be 14 stone [90 kilos], wasted away to six stone [38 kilos] and was no longer capable of making any decisions for himself. While the big fellow in the corner could no longer speak and had no idea what was going on. I was the only one of the four that walked out of the hospital some six or seven days later in any reasonable state of health at all. Diabetes does take over your life, and when you see these other serious instances it does focus the mind. It's something that you live with every single day.

Margo and I try to go the Art Gallery of New South Wales every Thursday to hear a lecture at 1 p.m., but every Thursday at 10 a.m., when I'm doing my reading, I have to tell her whether I'm up to going in or not—because if I'm 12+ mmol/L forget it. If I'm under, say 10, with a bit of luck I'll get by, so long as I don't go hypo before lunch. So I have to organise the attendance at the lecture and my morning tea and my breakfast so that I can eat before I go into the lecture so I don't go hypo in the lecture.

Tim: I guess you can't start eating in the lecture?

Geoff: I can't step outside of the house without taking a food pack. Any time I'm going out I take two sandwiches with peanut butter, one apple or one mandarin and a pocket full of glucose, and I've got to eat regularly. I might go to the hairdressers and I'll say, 'Joe hang on a minute, I've got to eat a sandwich and an apple'.

'You've got to eat a sandwich?'

And I say, 'Yes, my haircut takes fifteen minutes and I'm going a bit low, I might get a bit sick'.

'You look alright to me!'

'Yes', I say, 'this is the irony of diabetes'.

I've had it said to me a number of times: 'For somebody who claims to be as sick as you are, you're the healthiest looking man I've ever seen.' But you don't see me when I'm sick because I'm in hospital and you're not visiting me. You don't see me when I'm lying at home on the sofa or in bed, you're not there observing that. You observe me when I know I am capable of going out. Then I'm okay, that is with a reading between 4 and 8. Under those circumstances you've got colour in your face, you're okay. So I walk with a bit of a limp—well most people over 60 walk with a bit of a limp, no big deal. You don't see me when I'm sweating on a cold winter's day because I'm having an epileptic fit. You don't see me when I've fallen on one leg in the Domain, walking up to Wynyard from the Art Gallery, because I've gone hypo and Margo's unwrapping four glucose tablets to put in my mouth. You don't see that. You only see me when I'm of the view that I'm able to be seen.

Tim: What did the barber say to that?

Geoff: No one knows what you're talking about. They don't know what diabetes is. Occasionally they'll see a little story on the television—children at Newcastle, one a day going into hospital etc. Their kids don't have diabetes, they're not listening, they're cooking dinner. They don't see the dysfunctional consequences, the adverse effects because we hide that from people, don't we. I've cancelled doctor's appointments because I can't go. Margo and I have signed up for 30 lectures at the Art Gallery this year—we've had

> 20 and I've missed about four. A piano recital I was supposed to go to at Angel Place about three weeks ago, I couldn't go because my readings were so low at 6 p.m., I thought this is not a goer. I keep giving tickets to Margo to go to performances I've booked. The people I sit next to never see me when I'm ill on the nights I can't attend. They only see me when I'm there and I'm on top of my act. They don't see the downside—they only see me when I'm looking good. When I'm fit enough to hop into the ring with Mike Tyson and go three rounds.

Geoff is the hidden face of Type 2 diabetes, the man who drew one of the shortest of all the diabetic straws. I felt guilty about my own, by comparison, rude health. He was nice enough not to be resentful—or to show resentment to me anyway. Geoff is a polite and civilised man. I often think about him. Alas, there *is* no justice in matters of health. Perhaps when he progresses to insulin, he will find his diabetes easier to control. I certainly hope so. He deserves a break!

As Geoff himself is quick to point out, his case is 'atypical'. Perhaps a relief to the rest of us recently diagnosed members of the diabetic club, but cold comfort to him. However, he refuses to buckle under to his medical problems. He manages to take a piano lesson every week, practises daily and sits (and passes) exams. Geoff is studying Latin with the University of Sydney Continuing Education program, reads serious literature, follows the stock market and subscribes to the opera, ballet and theatre.

'Some days I don't make the grade, but in many more ways I do.'

(Just before this book went to press, I contacted Geoff to see how he was going. There was some good news for a change.

His diabetes had stabilised and he was getting 'an excellent set of statistics', although his somewhat gloomy physician cautioned him that he was probably 'only in a holding pattern'! Geoff and Margo have booked themselves on a cruise around the South Pacific, which wouldn't have been an option when we first spoke.)

So let me quickly give you two more examples of people with Type 2 diabetes who have admittedly had better luck than Geoff, but who have also tackled the condition forthrightly, refusing to let it dominate their lives.

Michael Plutte is an export manager in the field of gourmet food—a difficult area in which to keep svelte, and he isn't. He's now had Type 2 diabetes for ten years, and was diagnosed at age 54 during a routine health check-up. At 125 kilos Michael knew he was obese, but exercised regularly—swimming and gym workouts—even before he was diagnosed. He lost 20 kilos at one stage, but put it all back on. 'More recently I'm losing it again by a low-carbohydrate diet and zero alcohol,' he told me.

He did not, and has not, joined Diabetes Australia, nor been to any public health lectures or forums. But he has managed to find out the information he thought he needed from other sources. Michael sees his GP 'as rarely as possible', and has his eyes and feet checked 'when I am reminded'.

Being in the food business he is savvy about what he should be eating. Despite the extra weight he's carrying he has been able to control his diabetes without drugs for the past ten years. Michael is optimistic about his future health. We corresponded by email and I asked him if he thought about diabetes much?

'Only when you ask me all these questions! For me, it's no

big deal. I get on with my life, am aware of what I eat, and exercise regularly.'

Richard, like me, has only recently been diagnosed. He is a sales director with an optical company and was picked up at the age of 59 in a routine medical check-up. He was surprised to be told he had Type 2 diabetes and did not know of any family members with the disease:

> Once the diagnosis was confirmed by the glucose test I decided to instantly change my diet and adopt an exercise program. I was surprised to learn that diabetes could not be cured, but my doctor convinced me that if I changed my habits I would not need medication, at least for some time. I have not had a chocolate, ice cream or eaten any sweet items from that moment. No exceptions! I started walking and then jogging—but knocked my feet about so went back to brisk walking the next day.

Richard did join Diabetes Australia, but like Michael, was not attracted to any group activity. He managed to bring his blood glucose levels back down to between 6 and 8 mmol/L within three months. He has some friends who are Type 1 and only one who is Type 2:

> He is hopeless. He eats puddings with ice cream and drinks lots of full-strength beer, along with whisky and Coke! He was jetted out of Broome last year to Adelaide and had his little toe and part of his foot amputated. He is my inspiration!

By contrast to his friend, Richard is Spartan. Weather permitting he walks for 45 minutes each morning before breakfast, and a longer walk during the weekend. He watches his low-fat, low-carbohydrate diet carefully. 'I do not relent or "treat" myself.' He has brought his weight down from 100 to 90 kilos, but like me has not yet managed an alcohol-free day:

> I have cut out full-strength beer and only drink low-strength beer occasionally—for example, while camping and driving at Cape York! I stick almost exclusively to red and white wine, but no 'sticky' whites any more.

Richard has annual eye and feet check-ups, and is controlling his diabetes with diet and exercise. He is optimistic about leading a normal healthy life—'possibly healthier, in fact'.

With GPs the first port of call for most people diagnosed with Type 2, it is perhaps not surprising to learn that this experience is like the famous curate's egg—good in parts. I was fortunate to be picked up early in my progression into Type 2 by a GP who encounters the condition in some 20 per cent of his patients. Yet I talked to a number of people who had less than satisfactory experiences with their local doctors. I decided to explore the difficulties facing patients and GPs with this sometimes hard-to-spot disease.

Dr Ian Adair is the Chief Executive Officer of the Alliance of NSW Divisions in Sydney—an organisation which promotes the work of the NSW Divisions of General Practice. Among its many functions the Alliance works closely with health planners, health professionals, consumers and state and federal health bureaucracies.

Tim: Can Type 2 diabetes be hard to recognise?

Ian: It can be. Diagnosis can often be clouded by other presenting issues. I guess I'd also have to say that there are bound to be a group of GPs—and specialists for that matter—

who are not particularly sensitive to the issue, and that's true for all professions across the spectrum of their activities. Often the problem in general practice is that someone can come to their doctor with a list of symptoms that can be far from crystal clear. The situation can be clouded by other issues—and you have quoted several examples. For instance, frequent urination on its own is not necessarily a pointer to diabetes. There is the classic triad of symptoms—an increased appetite, increased thirst and increased urination. But if you don't have all of those present, and might have a fever combined with a burning sensation when you pass urine, then it can be more complicated.

Tim: With men it could be prostate problems?

Ian: Well frequency of urination could be prostate. If it's someone younger and they are sexually active it could be a urinary tract infection—particularly if it's a woman. If you are feverish you get thirsty and you may also get hungry unless you are feeling physically unwell, in which case you would lose your appetite. So there are some complications in the diagnostic process. That said, it should be on the list of things a doctor considers at the time in the absence of symptoms or signs of anything else. In the absence of any other sign of infection or disease, you should be thinking diabetes. I think most GPs, given five seconds to think about it, would be thinking that. GPs are particularly well placed generally as they often know the patient's family and personal history, which may include a history of diabetes.

That's not to say that errors don't happen, because they do. A patient should be told to come back in a couple of days if they don't improve. But do they, even if they are told that? I know from my own experience people do not always come back when they're told to. So the question then becomes, 'Well what's the contribution of the patient? Don't patients have a responsibility to look after their own health as well?'

Tim: Do you think that GPs test patients enough for blood glucose?

Ian: That raises a very interesting point because, unless I'm mistaken, the tolerance for blood glucose has actually dropped over the years. In other words, what was an acceptable upper limit has actually fallen. The same thing has happened with blood pressure. When I started as a medical student an acceptable blood pressure was 100 plus your age on 90. When I graduated it was 160 on 90. By the time I went into general practice people were starting to get worried when it was 150. Then when I came into general practice for a second time it was 140 on 90. Today you're looking at 130 on 80. So the tolerance levels for these sorts of things have shrunk with time as better information becomes available. You mention in your book about diet and whether simple sugars are the cause and the great evil of diabetes, or whether it is just part of a broader picture. That was the accepted wisdom 30, 20 or even 10 years ago, and that was certainly what I was taught in medical school—that simple sugars were the great no-no in diabetes. So it's not surprising that doctors of all types—specialists included—who aren't specialists in that area, still have that background impression unless they have been told otherwise.

Now the focus on the glycaemic index is really only something that has come out in the last five years, certainly in a major way.

Tim: What about the case of Geoff who went to an older GP, who told him to test his blood glucose by piddling on test strips that hadn't been used for 20 years or so?

Ian: There are certainly some older GPs around who have not kept up with continuing medical education or the information available to them has not been across a sufficient range of topics to keep them abreast of relatively common conditions and their management. I think there are a couple of things that are happening at the moment that have an impact on this. One is that the emphasis on education and continuing education is increasing for doctors. I think that one of the great problems with it, one of the difficulties in general practice, is the sheer range of topics that you have to be able to cover. And that sometimes leads to an unfortunate situation where community expectations exceed the practical capacity of a GP to satisfy. That's not an indication, necessarily, for people to launch off and go to a specialist. The onus is on the GP to have sufficient knowledge to be able to identify a problem, and once identifying it, if they don't feel confident, then they should refer. What sometimes happens is that some GPs—and I truly believe this is only a tiny minority—operate outside their sphere of competence. But that's true of specialists too. There are plenty of specialists' disaster stories around too.

And I think that part of the role of medical organisations should be to encourage two things: competence within the profession itself but also encouraging patients to take responsibility when they believe there is something wrong. To give them the confidence to say to their doctor, 'Look I don't agree, this doesn't feel right. I ought to go somewhere else'. Too many patients lack the confidence to say to their doctor, 'You will have to explain more because I don't feel comfortable with this'. Or even say, 'I just don't believe you—prove it to me!'

Tim: Do you think there are significant differences between the diagnosis of Type 2 diabetes by city GPs and those in the bush?

Ian: I think there is a very clear association between the time spent with a patient and the quality of both the diagnosis and the management. There is no evidence at all that you can give people the same amount of information in five minutes as you can in fifteen. It raises the issue of bulk-billing medical centres. I don't know whether the unfortunate Geoff, whom you interviewed, went to one of those or just picked up a slack GP—I have insufficient information to make the call. And not all bulk-billing medical centres have slack GPs in them either. It's almost like a generational change in general practice and a stratification of practice profile now between bulk billing—what you might call the McDonald's style of medicine—and the smaller corner store approach. All kinds of things happen in what amounts to a marketplace. However, there does seem to be a quality issue with high-volume practices, whether they be the big medical centre or the small corner store or one that just happens to be high on throughput.

I guess that's the reason why the College of General Practitioners has wanted to emphasise the benefits of longer consultations, particularly for complex problems. Almost by definition a problem that doesn't go away is a complex problem. It's certainly a chronic one after the first couple of months. So if someone is complaining that they are thirsty and they are always hungry and they are passing lots of urine—these are obvious things that might lead the GP to diagnose diabetes. But if they present primarily with, say, blurred vision or something else like tingling down one arm, even if they have diabetes, initially the diagnosis of diabetes will not be clear. For example, they might have just dislocated their shoulder so they have tingling down their arm. But if the shoulder is better and the tingling is still happening then the GP would have to be thinking about something else. Diabetes may be an incidental finding, or it may have caused the unsteadiness that led to the fall that caused the dislocation. The diagnosis may be completely different—it may be heart disease, with or without diabetes. If you don't stop and ask questions—which takes time—you're not going to find out what's wrong.

Tim: What role do you think the general practitioner should play in promoting public health?

Ian: Our view on this, not fully formed yet, is that general practice should be moving more towards the management of wellness and the maintenance of wellness, rather than simply treating illness when it occurs. What we are trying to do, and what we want to do—and we are under no illusions that it is probably going to take 10 to 20 years to do it—is to try and shift the mindset of our members that way. As one of our rural guys pointed out recently, if you have 2000 people knocking on your door because you are the only doctor for 2000 people, it is a lot harder to focus on wellness instead of the cuts and the skin cancers and whatever emergencies come through the surgery door. But unless we try and move towards such a policy, chronic illnesses such as diabetes are only going to increase.

Tim: So do you think GPs are aware enough of Type 2 diabetes?

Ian: Generally yes—but with the proviso that 'you can lead a horse to water but you can't make it drink'. And some doctors will not, for whatever reason, have diabetes as an area of interest. Perhaps they may not see it as a major issue for whatever personal reason . . . but I think most are, and some are, 'afficionados', and can be almost as good as the best endocrinologist in managing Type 1 and Type 2, because they have a special interest in the area.

It is a really broad spectrum, and goes back to the comment I made earlier, which was that if someone is really concerned that they have Type 2 diabetes because it's in the family and they have some of the symptoms and signs of it, and they are not getting satisfaction from their current GP, then they probably need a second opinion. Or they should go back to that GP and say, 'Look I've got a family history, I'm eating too much, I'm putting on weight, I'm feeling lethargic, and I'm peeing too much. I think I've got diabetes because that is exactly what happened to my father'. Then it would be a singular GP who ignored that, and if they did, I would be recommending that they went somewhere else for their diabetes care. It may be that this particular doctor might be really crash hot on heart disease and the patient might also have angina and high blood pressure, which is being exceptionally well managed. They might just have this blind spot about diabetes. Then the patient may need to go on to an endocrinologist for that component of their care.

Tim: Some people might think it impertinent to suggest a diagnosis to their GP?

Ian: I think we are all wary of people who come to doctors with a wad of papers off the Internet—but even that demonstrates that there is a measure of concern about an aspect of their health which has caused them to spend some hours looking it up. So the GP should take it seriously. If someone comes in with a stack of papers about diabetes and a family history of it and they have symptoms of it themselves, then that is a legitimate concern. As far as diabetes is concerned, the diagnostic test is easily done, and is a comparatively cheap one in the total scheme of things. If the BGL is normal they can be reassured; if not, then the GP and his or her patient can work together to manage the disease. Either way you have a good outcome.

Tim: I suppose people have to learn to be assertive if they really think there is something wrong with them, and also understand that the ceiling won't fall in if they tell their GP they want a second opinion.

Ian: That's right. And the same applies to lawyers or accountants for that matter.

Tim: Of course—but not journalists!

Ian: Oh of course not!

The brutal truth is that people with diabetes have to take control of their own disease. No one can do it for you. My GP, Ron, is quite adamant about that:

> I'm here to guide and help my patients if they want it. After I've asked someone if they would stop smoking two or three times—government people and other experts say you should bring it up every time they come in—I don't bother. I say to people on the second or third episode, 'When you're ready to give up let me know'. Because it can only work if they're ready to do it. It's the same with drinking. Someone is diabetic and they're drinking eight schooners a day. If they don't want to change that, there's not much I can do. I can tell them what's

going to happen if they don't—the likelihood of early heart attacks, strokes and so on—but that's about as far as I can go.

Quite a number of people don't want to change their lifestyle. However, even moderate changes can make a big difference to a person with diabetes. But if the patient doesn't want to change—it's their choice in the end.

CHAPTER FIVE

The silent assassins

One of the most insidious qualities of Type 2 diabetes is that half the people who have it, don't know they've got it. In its early stages there are no symptoms. When these develop, sometimes after many years, considerable damage may have been done.

The main home monitoring test for diabetes is to check daily for levels of glucose in the blood. Saturated fats, however, do not show up on glucometer tests, and they are bad news for everyone, but particularly so for people with diabetes. In fact, blood fats are not monitored on a daily or even weekly level. Recommended screening for blood cholesterol and triglyceride levels is annual, more often only if they are abnormal. But because they don't present any quick, obvious symptoms, they are easy to ignore. This is unwise. According to Diabetes Australia–NSW dietitian, Alan Barclay, high cholesterol and triglyceride levels are implicated in heart attacks and strokes—the leading killers of people with diabetes:

Alan: People don't usually die of high blood glucose levels per se; it's the blocked arteries or cardiovascular complications that usually end up getting them one way or another. So it is absolutely essential to control blood pressure and blood fat levels to reduce the cardiovascular risk. A low saturated fat diet is recommended. It is important too, to reduce total fat intake because weight loss is also usually an issue for someone with Type 2 diabetes. In most cases, people with Type 2 diabetes tend to carry too much weight around the tummy. If you can lose some of that weight—the evidence suggests 5 to 10 per cent of your body weight, particularly from around your middle, reduces your 'insulin resistance', which is a feature of Type 2 diabetes—that will definitely help your blood glucose levels and usually blood pressure and blood cholesterol come down as well.

Tim: Which assists the body to cope with the diabetes?

Alan: Well, yes. There was a prospective diabetes study done in the United Kingdom, where they looked at a group of people with Type 2 diabetes and followed them up for a couple of decades. They provided, what was at the time, the best care as far as nutritional advice, physical activity and medications available, and saw what the outcomes were as they followed the participants over several decades. Blood glucose accounted for about a third of the risk of developing the complications. Blood cholesterol accounted for about a third. And blood pressure accounted for about a third.

Sure, diabetes is characterised by excessive glucose in the blood and excessive urination is because of that, but as far as the overall burden of the disease it's equally important to manage your blood cholesterol and triglyceride levels as well as your blood pressure. Usually if you can get weight down and have a good healthy diet and regular exercise, blood pressure and cholesterol levels improve as well as the blood glucose. Importantly HDL (good cholesterol) increases and LDL (bad cholesterol) decreases, as do the triglycerides.

Unfortunately many health professionals still fixate only on blood glucose levels, which may only cause one third of the possible damage to their patients, as Alan Barclay points out:

> Sometimes Type 2 diabetes patients are told to 'avoid all sugar and she'll be right mate'. Of course that is patently untrue: I guess almost 30 years of research has proven quite conclusively that sugar itself does not cause diabetes and nor is it necessary to avoid it completely in the management of diabetes. Often people start off on a bad foot, I think, when they get diagnosed and are told to avoid sugar totally and perhaps not much more—although I do believe that is changing, particularly over the past year or so.
>
> Perhaps Diabetes Australia can claim some credit there, because of the GI [glycaemic index] symbol program that we launched in July 2003 and, in particular, books such as *The New Glucose Revolution* and its stablemates, which have been around for about eight years now and certainly have captured the imagination of the public and helped enlighten health professionals. I think people are starting to let go of that 'avoid all sugar' model.

As someone with Type 2 diabetes I find it astonishing that fundamental knowledge about how best to treat Type 2 diabetes has changed so drastically in fairly recent times. For example, it wasn't until the 1970s that carbohydrates—bread, potatoes, grains, cereals and rice—were recognised as being an essential and good part of the diet of people with diabetes. Previously, carbohydrates had been demonised because they are processed into glucose—sugar—by our bodies. But without this essential fuel, we can't function properly. Our brains, in particular, must have glucose. So while glucose fuels our muscles, it can also cause blood glucose levels to rise in people with diabetes. Consequently, while carbohydrates are essential, they have to be eaten with care and knowledge.

What has been termed the 'GI revolution' is another recent development on the diabetic management scene. Carbohydrates, which are absorbed more slowly over a longer period of time, avoiding the damaging 'spikes' of high blood sugar immediately after a meal, are a useful tool in controlling diabetes. The GI, using a scale of 1 to 100, identifies the carbohydrates with best—or lowest—GI rating. Under 55 is deemed to be good, and those rating in the 30s and 40s are even better. More on the positive effects of GI later—but first some more bad news.

With one out of four Australians either in the pre-diabetic stage of glucose intolerance or with Type 2 diabetes—and only half of those aware of their situation—our fondness for fatty foods, takeaways and the inevitable increase in our waistlines are leading to a public health crisis of staggering proportions. Some would say it is already here.

Type 2 diabetes is estimated to cost Australia $3 billion a year. The average cost of a person with Type 2 diabetes, with no complications, is estimated at $10 900 a year. If there are complications, this doubles to $20 525. Diabetes Australia estimates that four per cent of people diagnosed with diabetes account for 12 per cent of the health costs in Australia. But these figures don't tell the whole story because of the cardiovascular complications. A heart bypass, for example, costs $80 000 to $100 000. It is believed that six out of ten people with diabetes will die of a heart attack or stroke. If you take into account amputations, kidney dialysis or heart operations, $3 billion a year is conservative. There are 3000 amputations a year because of diabetes—eight a day—and each one costs approximately $50 000. Then there are rehabilitation costs on top of that. Kidney dialysis is about $75 000 a year for each individual and up to half of the people on machines in hospitals around Australia are there because of diabetes.

A person with diabetes goes to the doctor more often, is hospitalised more often and will have a shorter life expectancy than the person who doesn't have diabetes. The reality is that the health budget is straining under the cost of diabetes care already. How will it cope in 20 years time?

Just blame our genes

So why does diabetes create such a public health crisis worldwide? Our genes are more than partly responsible. Humans had to survive a number of ice ages over the past 700 000 years. Huddling in chilly caves, our ancestors weren't able to grow crops, even if they knew how to do it. Through necessity they killed whatever animals they could, and survived on meat—essentially a high-protein diet. Paradoxically, this favoured those individuals who had insulin resistance. When there isn't much carbohydrate, the body copes by making sure the brain receives what little glucose there is, followed by the muscles. So these people survived better than the individuals who would have been deemed more healthy by today's standards, those able to process the carbohydrates they weren't getting!

Due to natural selection, however, we tend to be descended from the successful carnivore-eating, insulin-resistant ancestors. When the last ice age retreated and humans started growing fixed crops, such as cereal grains, vegetables and beans, their blood sugars shot up after eating because their ancestors had adapted, through necessity, to a high-protein diet.

Things got worse after the industrial revolution. New milling techniques encouraged mass-produced, highly refined carbohydrates, which actually increased the GI of what would have been a lower GI food naturally. Today, the supermarket revolution has unleashed a cornucopia of highly processed fatty and sugary foods, which we gobble up without any thought—not to mention the equally evil fast foods from fat and salt-laden pizzas to greasy burgers and big buckets of deep-fried chips. Faced with this glucose and saturated fat overload, the body frantically puts out more insulin from those splendidly named Islets of Langerhans in the pancreas. If a person teetering on the edge of diabetes is also overweight, the spare tyre of excess fat inhibits the ability of this extra insulin to control blood glucose levels. It's a vicious cycle. The pancreas works harder, the insulin can't do its job, blood sugars rise, and eventually the body's insulin supply starts to give out and . . . presto!—Type 2 diabetes.

European people, with three and four thousand years of settled agricultural settlement behind them, have had more time to adapt, genetically, to processing carbohydrates. A Harvard University study, involving thousands of men and women over many years, has shown that people who eat mostly refined foods with a high GI were two or three more times more likely to develop Type 2 diabetes or heart disease. Other races, such as native North Americans, Pacific Islanders and our own Australian Aborigines, were well adapted to their hunter–gatherer diets, but not to white bread, fast food and alcohol. The incidence of diabetes in some of these groups is, would you believe, as high as one adult in three. Recently a number of Australian Aboriginal people with diabetes were encouraged to return to a 'bush tucker' diet for a trial study. Their high blood sugar levels quickly dropped to normal. Urban living is a health hazard for everyone!

People diagnosed with diabetes have to be very careful about what they eat. So I started to be sensible about diet only after I'd been alerted to an incurable condition that will shorten my life in nasty ways if I didn't take note of what I was shoving into my mouth. Now I look about me as young—and perhaps not so young—grossly overweight people stuff themselves with greasy chips, pies and luridly coloured vanilla slices (God, how I loved them!), and swig over-sugared soft drinks as well as buckets of booze and feel I should shout out a warning! I'm in danger of becoming a health bore, so help me. But then again, like most people, I thought I was bulletproof in the health department.

Living in the dark

Let's again consider the fact that one out of two people with Type 2 diabetes, or insulin resistance, is unaware of their condition. They may have no symptoms for years. The high blood glucose levels of undiagnosed diabetics are remorselessly destroying the networks of fine capillaries in the body, which heroically help to filter and cleanse impurities from our blood.

Our kidneys have hundreds and thousands of these, and they keep on doing their job for years and years, although age itself has a negative effect. Many of these undiagnosed diabetics will also be smokers, which further damages the small blood capillaries that can never be replaced when they are gone. Kidney complications brought on under these circumstances are called diabetic nephropathy.

I was shocked to hear recently at a renal seminar I attended that people can lose 90 per cent of their kidney function—by which time they are close to complete and irreversible kidney failure—with virtually no symptoms. Unless a specific urine test is performed for a leakage of albumin into the urine—a microalbumin test—progressive kidney failure may not be detected early enough. Once the kidneys have failed, the only alternative is dialysis or a kidney transplant.

Many undiagnosed people with diabetes first seek medical help because they have problems with their eyes or feet. With consistently high blood sugar, the small blood vessels carrying oxygen and nutrients to the back of the eye—the retina—become blocked. New, but fragile, blood vessels may form to replace them, but are likely to break and bleed. Again, as is often the case with complications due to diabetes, there are no symptoms, and vision remains normal for quite some time. But this can be picked up by an ophthalmologist or an optician, who can look into the back of the eye with special instruments—which is why all people with Type 2 diabetes are encouraged to have eye checks at diagnosis, and then twice a year. Once there is damage then examination may need to be more often.

In cases where people are simply not aware of their diabetes, blood vessel damage at the back of the eye just goes on and on, and high blood pressure can increase this. Then there can be permanent scarring of the retina. The first indication of this can be a sudden partial loss of vision, which causes a visit to an ophthalmologist and often leads on to a diagnosis of diabetes. Fortunately, if there is an upside, if the diabetes is undiagnosed but the blood glucose levels are high, people often experience blurred vision which may then lead them to see an optometrist. The blurred vision is due to a change in the shape of the lens in the eye and is reversible when blood glucose levels are controlled. Laser therapy can be used to treat already damaged areas of the eye, and prevent further deterioration. But long-term damage cannot be reversed.

Another warning sign for people who aren't aware they have diabetes is numbness, or a burning feeling, or pins and needles in the feet—particularly at night in bed. This is caused by high blood glucose levels leading to nerve damage, particularly in the feet—diabetic peripheral neuropathy. Because numb feet are more liable to be injured, fairly severe damage can be done, for example, by hot water bottles or even a stone in a shoe. Cracked heels may allow infections to occur and some people may develop callouses and even ulcers from too much pressure on some areas of their feet. Sometimes toes or legs have to be amputated, particularly in feet which have a loss of sensation or reduced blood supply. Heavy drinking can contribute to diabetic neuropathy—worse luck! People with diabetes are urged to have their feet checked by a podiatrist at least once a year.

And now it may be people's hearing that is affected by diabetes too. Recent research in the United States has pointed to premature ageing of the body's hearing system.

To continue my catalogue of gloom, I must also mention that undiagnosed diabetes will often be associated with raised blood pressure, leading to heart failure, heart attacks or strokes.

Diabetes will also add to atherosclerosis—the thickening and narrowing of the large arteries in the body—which happens to us all as we get older. The major causes of the narrowing of arteries in this area are smoking, high blood pressure, a high cholesterol level, high triglyceride levels, obesity, a family history of heart disease and lack of exercise.

Everyone knows that smoking is bad in almost every conceivable way for human health, but if someone with diabetes keeps smoking you'd have to say they have a particularly well-developed death wish. I've seen photographs of double amputees, who lost their legs because of smoking, sitting in their wheelchairs still puffing away . . .

Complications of diabetes

Diabetes and eye disease

Diabetic retinopathy is the leading cause of blindness in Australians under 60 years of age. The development of retinopathy is strongly related to the length of time diabetes has been present and the degree of blood glucose control. Regular checks and treatment can prevent retinopathy-caused blindness.

Diabetes and kidney disease

Diabetes is the second most common cause of end-stage renal disease (ESRD). In 2001, Type 1 and Type 2 diabetes accounted for 25 per cent (Type 1: 4 per cent, Type 2: 21 per cent) of all new cases of ESRD diagnosed in Australia.

Diabetes and lower limbs

Neuropathy or peripheral nerve disease and vascular damage may lead to leg ulcers and serious foot problems from which limb amputation may result.

Diabetes and heart disease/strokes

Diabetes is often associated with high blood pressure and high blood fats (cholesterol and triglycerides), which cause an increased risk of heart attacks and strokes.

The results of the Australian Diabetes, Obesity and Life Study (AusDiab) released April 2001 show that nearly one in four Australian adults has either diabetes or impaired glucose metabolism, both of which are associated with substantial increased risk of both diabetes and heart disease. Here are some sobering statistics.

- Diabetes is the sixth highest cause of death by disease in Australia.
- People with diabetes are almost three times more likely to have high blood pressure, obesity or elevated blood fats, e.g. cholesterol.
- They are two to three times more likely to have cardiovascular disease, e.g. heart disease and stroke.
- 65 to 80 per cent of people with diabetes will die of coronary heart disease.
- 15 per cent of people with diabetes have heart disease compared to 2.5 per cent without diabetes.
- Renal disease accounts for 8 to 14 per cent of deaths in people with diabetes.
- 5 per cent of people with diabetes will experience foot ulcers.
- Of the 3000 amputations each year in people with diabetes, most would have been preventable.

- Australia's indigenous population suffers the fourth highest rate of Type 2 diabetes in the world.

Courtesy of Diabetes Australia

Don't slit your wrists—yet!

While the consequences of undiagnosed diabetes are nasty, the news gets better (and it would need to!) for people who realise what is happening to them and begin taking their Type 2 diabetes seriously. Sure, there is no cure as such, but knowledge about how to control diabetes with diet, exercise and medication enables many of us with Type 2 diabetes to get on with our lives with excellent prospects of having long and healthy futures.

When I got my wakeup call, I lost ten kilos (and should attempt a few more), began a regular exercise program of walking and cycling and adopted a low-fat, low-sugar diet—and even cut back on my enthusiastic wine consumption. Ron, my GP, assisted this process not only with advice, but by putting me on ACE inhibitor tablets (which contain, I'm told, an angiotensin converting enzyme) to lower my blood pressure (it also has beneficial side effects on kidney performance as well as the cardiovascular system) and increasing my daily cholesterol-lowering tablet (one of the group of drugs known as statins) from 10 to 20 mg. Apart from vitamins—and a low-dose aspirin—they are the only drugs I take.

(I was fascinated to hear that the liver controls 90 per cent of the release of cholesterol into the body. So if you are genetically predisposed to high cholesterol levels, there is a limit to what you can do to lower your blood fats by dieting. As my GP, Ron, put it in his inimitable style: 'People eat grass for a month and then find their cholesterol has only come down less than a percentage point.' Unless you take the pills, cholesterol levels will remain unacceptably high—certainly for those with diabetes. *Statins* do a much better job—although taking the pills and then getting stuck into King Island double cream and soft cheeses is *not* recommended.)

None of these drugs I'm on are specifically for Type 2 diabetes as I have managed to get my blood glucose levels (BGL) back to within the normal range, between 4 and 8 mmol/L. However, because I have progressed to Type 2 diabetes, the morning fasting readings are often higher than normal.

Because my condition was picked up early—although I must have been in the insulin-resistant phase for perhaps a year or two beforehand—my kidneys are fine, my valiant liver has breathed a sigh of relief at having to process less alcohol, and my eyes have not been affected by retinopathy. I've been a bit remiss in not having my feet checked yet, but I'm going to do that very soon. If I continue to live in a healthy way—and let's face it, *everyone* would be better off on a diabetic regime—I should be able to keep my blood sugars within the 'normal' range 'for some years yet', Ron thinks. That is as far as he will commit.

The next step for me, when my hard-working pancreas can no longer provide enough insulin without help, will be medication to lower blood glucose. It's all a matter of time really. Because I was diagnosed in my mid sixties, I will *probably* drop off the twig before progressing from medication to insulin injections. If I had been diagnosed in my forties, it is more likely I would eventually have to inject insulin. But nothing is absolutely certain with diabetes. What *is* certain is that if I relax and start behaving as though I did not have the disease, it would certainly catch up with me.

It is time for some good news.

Assuming a diagnosis of Type 2 diabetes has been confirmed, early kidney damage, picked up by the microalbumin test, can be reversed. Kidneys really want to do an honest job for us, and will continue to do so with modest help. Providing blood pressure and LDL 'bad' cholesterol are lowered, cardiovascular risks are drastically reduced. Getting blood sugar levels back into the 'normal' range (between 4 and 8 mmol/L) will provide similar benefits, and also lessen the chances of eye damage (retinopathy) as well as loss of sensation or a burning feeling in feet (neuropathy). And, of course, regular exercise is essential to keep generally healthy, and to burn up glucose—providing you don't overdo it and cause a hypo! (This is a problem most likely to affect those taking insulin, or on some other types of medication, who have to be more careful juggling their glucose levels throughout the day than early-stagers like me.)

Recent studies in England have proved that if people with diabetes, through good management, can actually lower their HbA1c ratings by a percentage point—over 7 is bad news, 6 is normal—they will drastically improve their chances of avoiding strokes or a heart attack by as much as 30 per cent. Which is good news for those of us with Type 2 diabetes—so long as we do what we should do, and that is the critical part. All the best advice and treatment available to us in the whole wide world will be useless unless individuals take control of their own disease and, by doing so, their quality of life into the future.

Buoyed up with enthusiasm after achieving BGL figures that our ex-Labor Prime Minister and Treasurer Paul Keating (had he been aware of them) would have described as 'a beautiful set of numbers'—I put it to my GP, Ron, that perhaps I would be better off in the long term now that I'd stopped living like there was no tomorrow:

Tim: You told me when I was diagnosed that diabetes wasn't a death sentence, it was a life sentence?

Ron: Absolutely. In fact, you're going to do better now that you know you're a diabetic, than you would if you hadn't known, because you were picked up very, very early and you have done no damage. Your HbA1c has never been high and you've changed your lifestyle, your weight is down, you're much more conscious of your lifestyle, your alcohol intake, your exercise and so on, than you would have been. People need a shock. It's not just a matter of fixing your diabetes, you need to fix your lifestyle.

Tim: But when I say to you, 'Maybe it's a good thing, maybe I'll live longer now', you get vague on me?

Ron: Because no doctor can guarantee an individual is going to live longer. You could walk outside and get run over by a bus. It happens.

Tim: But isn't it theoretically possible that I might live longer because I've started to take good care of my health, even though I've got a chronic, incurable condition?

Ron: Absolutely, there's no doubt about that. Obviously we have to talk in statistical population groups but there's no doubt that if you do all the right things, you will live a lot longer unless you get some other disease. But from a diabetic, or vascular, point of view, the incidence of heart attack can be 25 to 30 per cent less for people who aren't diabetic. Now we all know heart attacks can kill you. A recent study has shown that if you can reduce your HbA1c rating just by 0.9 per cent there are enormous benefits. That's been studied over ten years with control groups, and even people who only achieved a 0.7 per cent lower level in their HbA1c rating had a 25 per cent less chance of heart attacks—which is very encouraging.

Tim: What about people who go into denial and refuse to acknowledge their Type 2 diabetes?

Ron: That's common too—especially in people who drink a lot of alcohol and refuse to give that up. If you drink heavily, you really can't control diabetes.

Tim: What is it about alcohol and diabetes?

Ron: Mainly it's calorific—you tend to put on weight. When you drink moderately heavily, you lose your inhibitions and don't worry so much about what you eat. Instead of doing exercise, you're drinking. I'm not talking about people—like you Tim—who just have a few glasses of red wine, but really heavy drinkers.

I don't want to seem obsessed with the topic of alcohol—okay, well I am a journalist—but the prospect of not being able to have a few glasses of wine each day would be abysmal. However, I quickly discovered that there are some curious myths about alcohol and diabetes—for example, that beer should be avoided because it has more carbohydrate than wine, and that low-sugar beer is better for you.

All the 'how to' books on diabetes say you should not have more than two or three standard drinks a day, and if possible throw in a couple of alcohol-free days each week. I have always thought that a few glasses of red can only be beneficial. I was agreeably surprised when I talked about this with Alan Barclay, the dietitian at Diabetes Australia–NSW:

Alan: There's actually a benefit to people, if you've got Type 2 diabetes, in having some alcohol. It does improve insulin sensitivity and there are a vast number of studies that suggest that—but it's not going to be recommended as tonic!

Tim: A couple of glasses of red a day?

Alan: You're probably aware that the National Health and Medical Research Council have set their guidelines and they're founded on strong evidence. Alcohol consumption is the famous J-shaped curve that Mr Keating used to like to talk about, so those who have none at all are probably less healthy than those that have a little—who are much more healthy than those who have a lot. So this has been worked out and debated internationally, but in Australia it's one standard drink a day for women and two for men.

Tim: Standard drinks!—I don't know if you've ever had a standard drink—but it seems about the size of a thimble.

Alan: Especially with wine. We had a master's student a couple of years ago who did her thesis on this. The evidence is that to get the maximum benefit, you really only need one glass—a standard drink per day. Anything else is extra and will contribute to weight gain. It's all a matter of total calories really, and your body prefers to burn up alcohol first over other foods and this is what classically happens. This is where the myth of the beer belly comes from. You drink your beer and you have your fatty chips or your peanuts at the same time, your body metabolises the alcohol and will shunt the rest of the fat into storage. In men, of course, this is usually around the middle. That's the problem. You don't usually find overweight or obese alcoholics. In fact, if they die and an autopsy is done, their arteries are usually pretty clean because they're not eating anything at all. However, alcohol itself can cause low blood sugar, even in people who are not diabetic, because alcohol stops the liver from producing glucose, so people with diabetes who are on certain tablets to stimulate the pancreas to make more insulin, or are taking insulin, need to be aware of this and eat some carbohydrate while they are drinking.

The combination of the alcohol with the fatty foods has another problem. You can have hypos up to 36 hours after a drinking binge. Now if you're on insulin, that can be deadly, especially with Type 1. You've had too much to drink, you come home and just fall down into bed. If you don't have the food you should have and if you don't wake up at your usual time—and often if you've had too much to drink you don't want to get out of bed too early—it can literally be deadly. Obviously with someone with Type 2 who's on insulin, that risk is increased, and certainly with someone with tablets for Type 2 diabetes there's a risk also. There are definite dangers here.

In moderation, though, alcohol is certainly not a bad thing. One thing I have to constantly point out to most people is that there actually isn't a lot of sugar in any alcoholic drinks. There is a small difference between sweet or dry wines, but you're looking at about half a teaspoon of sugar per glass.

Tim: Beer I gather is pretty bad news?

Alan: No.

Tim: Really? It doesn't worry me so much, because I don't drink so much beer these days. But some people are passionate about their beer, and desolate when they can't have it because of their diabetes.

Alan: They're just ill-informed, unfortunately. There's no evidence that any form of alcohol is any better than the other. It's thought to be the alcohol molecule, per se, that has the benefits.

Tim: What about the carbohydrates in beer then?

Alan: Well there's hardly any.

Tim: This is good news!

Alan: Yes it is. I'd love to recruit some people to do some GI studies on alcohol, but we think that's not ethical. You'd have to drink so much to get the necessary 50 grams of carbohydrates on board—because there's hardly any carbs in beer—the researchers would be basically falling on their faces. There's about two and a half grams of sugar in 100 millilitres of beer, which is the total carbohydrate. Obviously you'd drink more beer than you would wine, but there are similar quantities of sugar in wine. Some brewers have actually produced low-sugar beers, but of course they're much higher in alcohol and they don't taste particularly good. The risk to the individual having a low-sugar beer is probably greater—for their overall health—than having a standard beer. It's the same with chocolate. I say have *one* real chocolate, your favourite one, and enjoy it. What's the point in having something you don't like? You might as well have one of your favourite beers and enjoy every mouthful than two of the ones that are lower in sugar, thinking you're doing yourself a favour—you're not.

Warning signals for diabetes

Symptoms can include:

- thirst and higher than normal urination
- unexplained periods of weakness and fatigue
- periods of blurred vision
- skin infections
- tingling and numbness in feet
- slow healing.

There may be no symptoms at all, so if you have a history of diabetes in your family, are overweight and don't do regular exercise—get yourself checked out!

And let's not forget about sex . . .

Like most aspects of diabetes, its effect on the sex lives of those who have it varies from the trivial to—well—disastrous. It is a complex situation that depends, to a great extent, on psychological as well as physiological factors. To be less discursive, a man who can't get an erection and is losing feeling in the important bits, or a women who is losing genital sensation or, paradoxically, feeling vaginal pain during intercourse because of diabetes-induced neuropathy, clearly need help if they can get it.

On the other hand, as we grow older, orgasmic sex for many couples seems less urgent and important than it once did. People may take great comfort and satisfaction from physical closeness, communication and intimacy that doesn't involve pole-vaulting around the room or swinging from the chandeliers (I have never managed this myself, even when young). A lot depends on what manner of sex life a couple were having before one of them became diabetic. It may well be that continuing enthusiasm overcomes whatever difficulties diabetes introduces to the equation. Or conversely, if there hasn't been a lot of action in the bedroom in past years, there aren't going to be any quick fixes with or without diabetes.

Diabetes can affect the blood flow into the hydraulic system of the penis that causes an erection. Any effects on the nerve system can also influence the mechanism which coordinates this blood flow. The result is an erection which is not firm enough for penetration, or does not last long enough for intercourse. Added to this is the psychological element of worry about performance—it might be a better use of time to switch on the bedside table lamps and get on with that good book.

If an erection is achieved, maintained, and got where it should be, diabetes can have another unpleasant surprise lurking in the mechanism. When nerves in the genital area are affected, it is possible for men to have dry orgasms—no ejaculation—a decreased intensity of orgasm, no orgasm at all or, most disappointing of all, an orgasm they can't feel at all. Under certain circumstances men may also have a kind of reverse ejaculation—it goes back into the bladder. This last one isn't all that much of a problem, more of a surprise, until the person concerned realises what is going on—it is also less messy!

So what can be done about erectile dysfunction?

There are various mechanical contrivances, splints and vacuum pumps, and also Viagra—and other fairly recently developed drugs—which can overcome these difficulties, if the spirit is also willing. There are also injections directly into the penis, some of which are reputed to induce utterly dependable, rock-hard erections for up to twenty-four hours—were I ever to come to this (so to speak) I wonder about the extent to which I could put this priapic splendour to adequate use? (I have a sneaking feeling my partner of 35 years might not feel quite so enthusiastic about such a marital marathon.)

There has been less research done on the sexual difficulties encountered by women with diabetes, than with men. What has been established is that women do suffer sexual dysfunction. This can include low sexual desire, orgasm difficulties and painful intercourse—although perhaps not significantly more than women without diabetes. In some studies there were more arousal difficulties than with non-diabetic women.

Professor Lesley Campbell, who heads the Diabetes Centre at St Vincent's Hospital in Sydney, and who enjoys a worldwide reputation in the field of diabetes research, has written in some detail about sexual difficulties encountered by people with diabetes in her excellent book *Understanding Diabetes*. The Diabetes Centre's own research, carried out in 1989, found that a woman's sexual satisfaction related to her pre-diabetes sexual history and relationship happiness, rather than to any particular problem arising from the diabetes:

Tim: I take it from what you say that men have received most of the research attention when it comes to diabetes and sex?

Lesley: Yes of course. It seems that wherever money is, that's where the drug companies fearlessly will go. Erectile dysfunction has become big . . .

Tim: As it were . . .

Lesley: Yes, big! We had a big public discussion day at the Garven Institute recently and I thought to myself that I *used* to do the sex talk and now I do the obesity talk—which must say something about my age I think. They get a nice young man to do the erectile dysfunction talk these days. As it happens I have written the only paper on female sexual dysfunction in Australia, which is the least quoted paper ever written. It's interesting how the emphasis on research into male sexuality has evolved. When I first started talking about that, there wasn't that much information available, except that there was nerve damage, which is quite common due to neuropathy. This can lead to autonomic nerve damage and there can be arterial blood supply damage as well.

Tim: Presumably with loss of sensation and loss of performance as well?

Lesley: An erection is an engineering marvel. You've not only got to have the thought, you've got to have this huge blood supply go there in a few moments. So you need a lot of blood diverting there and sort of staying there, and both of those things can go wrong. It's been taken over basically by the sexologists, the male counsellors; it's become really big stuff because there's so many treatments now. But it's mostly combined dysfunction.

It turned out that there wasn't just one thing that was to blame. Most men are fragile creatures emotionally it turns out, so if something didn't work out perfectly they became stressed and tense. The funny thing is that that is more likely to manifest as a problem with a girlfriend rather than a wife. It's alright when there is routine—this is hilarious, I learnt a lot about life during this particular research. So you don't malfunction with your wife because of the well-worn routine, but if you were with someone else, the inner voice keeps saying, 'It's got to work, it's got to work . . . ' and that's where the dysfunction is. I found that really fascinating. When the stress was on, that was the testing time, where performance anxiety kicked in.

Tim: What were some of the earlier treatments for lack of performance?

Lesley: One of the first things that was available for erectile dysfunction was a kind of vacuum device—which was really like a breast pump—which is still around. That used to pump up a vacuum so that the blood would engorge and then you just put a little band on at the base of the penis to hold the blood in there. It is non-toxic, though aesthetically not very exciting, as many who used it said. That was really all we had for a while. Then came injections, which are not unlike an insulin injection except it's a good idea not to mix them up!

The fascinating thing was that many of the men started with these techniques, but they had a high discontinuation rate; it was as though they wanted to know they *could* do it but not everybody went on doing it and quite a few people were anxious about it. Then came Viagra, and it had about a 60 to 70 per cent success rate. However, that was interesting from a psychological point of view, because the injections worked every time, but the Viagra still needed a message from the brain signalling desire to be effective.

Tim: It reminds me of the old joke: 'What is the lightest thing in the world? A penis, because a thought will raise it!'

Lesley: If it's working. So Viagra only works if you want it to and so do some of the new drugs. One turns your vision blue—there are a few side effects—and they're expensive too.

Tim: We've been talking about the mechanics of sex, but what about the emotional side?

Lesley: Let me give you an example. I had this one man who I referred on to a wonderful GP I use as a counsellor. Anyway, I never knew what the full psychology behind this was, but this man's wife stopped having sex with him after they had three children. Then 15 or 20 years passed with absolutely no action, and one day out of the blue she said to him, 'Okay, get on with it'! And of course he couldn't. So I sent him off to Margaret, the GP, and she said, 'Look, he doesn't want to'. That was the point. Why should he? And that was the counselling. The treatment was to *not* in fact give him Viagra, which wouldn't have worked, or to give him injections, which at the time was possibly all there was. What was the point of injecting it if he didn't want to? For 15 years, she didn't want any sex, so why should he suddenly spring into life?

Tim: What made her suddenly do that do you think?

Lesley: Possibly nasty motives. There were other things I didn't think were too good about this relationship.

Tim: A bit like, 'Perform, and if you can't that's something else I can hate you for'.

Lesley: Probably. Another time I did send someone to the urologist. Some people can't hold an erection because of a neurological thing called 'venous run-off'. They actually get an erection and it ebbs away. I asked the urologist to do these special tests—ghastly tests where they sort of fill the penis with saline, and they can tell if the saline runs away quickly that they've got this run-off. So I sent him off, very excited that I'd diagnosed this wonderful thing. Then the urologist contacted me saying, 'Alright, I'll do all your tests but the real reason he can't perform is he's married to the wrong woman'. I thought this wasn't the urologist's job to make those kind of assumptions, and said that I still wanted him to do the tests—which weren't conclusive. His hunch was probably the right one. In the end counselling is still part of the deal, you can't take the tests out of the context of the relationship.

Tim: So what about women, sex and diabetes?

Lesley: This is a fascinating area and still largely unresolved. The conclusion of our research paper was—and this is not a nice one for feminism I'm afraid—30 to 40 per cent of the Australian women we interviewed complained of loss of sexual satisfaction.

Tim: Not sexual desire, but sexual satisfaction?

Lesley: If you look for the counterpart of the erection, it is only lubrication—which can be fixed if they didn't have that. By the way I should say we didn't have a control group. Our advice at the time was diabetes shouldn't have been the cause of loss of lubrication, that it was just dissatisfaction. But I now think diabetes did have an effect.

Tim: Do you mean it stopped the lubrication?

Lesley: Well, as I said, if lubrication was a problem it's easy enough to fix, but these women were actually not getting satisfaction. They had been orgasmic and they now weren't and they weren't enjoying it. That's what they said. What I've heard anecdotally from women since that experiment is that it's happening to them. I've actually been able to detect them losing feeling—developing neuropathy. So I'm beginning to think that diabetes is the cause of that and somehow the neuropathy is causing those sexual problems, and I think other people are now finding that. But there's been so little investigation of women and so many studies of males. However, more work is being done now. They have even been trying to use Viagra in women but it's not working. Viagra works on blood vessels and dilating blood vessels, so the women aren't getting anywhere.

Tim: Wouldn't you say—I guess Rupert Murdoch must be an exception to this, siring children after prostate cancer at 70—that the sexual urge tends to drop off markedly for most people once they pass their sixties?

Lesley: Absolutely. Margaret Redelman, the GP that helped write the chapter on sex in *Understanding Diabetes*, makes the point that people don't recognise what age does. If they don't, they completely miss the point because that's one of the biggest things that affects sexuality. They often think that something's wrong with them, when that's the normal ageing process. Margaret says people can do other things, rather than conventional intercourse, and still enjoy themselves in their relationships. In life people have this picture in their minds, this dream of performance—perhaps exemplified by the 24-hour erection. But reality is, of course, quite different. The mistake is to carry that picture in the mind and think that's important. It's far more satisfying to explore areas of much more mutual personal interaction.

CHAPTER SIX

What can I eat?

'You are what you eat.' People with diabetes know full well the truth of this misquoted aphorism.[1] I am exceedingly fond of good tucker, and when I was diagnosed with Type 2 diabetes the prospect of a life-long dietary hair shirt was one of the spectres that preyed on my mind. A year on I'm a lot more cheerful about diet, and continually amazed at the huge range of delicious goodies that are available for members of the Type 2 club. In small servings of course!

It is bleedingly, blindingly, obvious that everyone on earth would be better off if they ate a diabetic diet—low saturated fat, low sugar, plenty of fruit and vegetables, fish and lean meat,

1 The French politician and legendary gastronome, Jean Anthelme Brillat-Savarin (1755–1826), originally coined the phrase, 'Tell me what you eat and I shall tell you what you are'. This was echoed by the philosopher, Ludwig Feurerbach, who was quoted in 1850 as saying, 'Man is what he eats'. This has morphed into the less gender specific, 'You are what you eat'.

wholegrain bread, more foods with a low GI (glycaemic index) and moderate alcohol intake. Not only that, public health would be vastly improved, hospital waiting lists would vanish, many GPs would have less business, the health budget could be halved, and we'd all live far past our allotted span of four score years and ten. And we might even find fairies at the bottom of the garden.

But life's not like that, is it?

Those with diabetes do have to be very careful about what they allow past their lips. In some respects this is more critical for Type 1 people, who have to eat small meals regularly throughout the day to balance their insulin injections to avoid hypers and hypos. Those with Type 2 are not on such a critical dietary tightrope. Even for Type 2 people who have progressed to injecting insulin, usually requiring only two injections a day—morning and evening—the pancreas is still producing some insulin, which avoids (mostly) the sudden peaks and troughs of their blood glucose levels. Which is where the GI is even more important—but more on that in a moment.

The low-down on carbohydrates

As previously mentioned, sugar is not the bogey it was once thought to be. It is just another form of carbohydrate, which we must have to survive. It has to be watched, of course, but one chocolate or an ice-cream isn't going to lop minutes off your life. In fact, low-fat ice-cream can be part of a healthy diet, and manufacturers make such a good job of it, that I can hardly tell the difference now. (But try and get it in small tubs! You can look in vain in freezer bins in garages and corner shops for portion-sized, low-fat ice-creams. It only seems to be available in big tubs in supermarkets. I'm going to take it up as a crusade!)

I find it interesting that food manufacturing companies have now detected that there is a profit to be made from advertising lower fat products, such as low-fat fruit yoghurts. Better labelling, detailing the fat content and GI of food, is a welcome advance. With obesity one of our biggest public health challenges, this admirable trend by the big food manufacturing companies seems destined to continue. Perhaps I'll even be able to buy a low-fat ice-cream from a servo before too long. (I am told one manufacturer has this in mind—but I'll believe it when I see it.) Stung by allegations that they only purvey junk food, big fast-food outlets like McDonald's are now advertising a range of vegetarian and low-fat 'healthy' takeaways.

We do need fats, of the right kind, to function properly. But saturated fats are the biggest no no. Before my diabetes was diagnosed I was only dimly aware of the distinction between saturated fats, polyunsaturated fats and mono-unsaturated fats (contained in olive and canola oil). Essentially people with Type 1 and Type 2 diabetes have to take an intelligent interest in what they eat. Their survival and long-term health depends on it.

Cholesterol and diabetes

There are two main kinds of cholesterol. Low density lipoprotein (LDL) cholesterol, which takes cholesterol from the liver into the rest of the body, depositing it in the blood vessels if levels get too high, and high density lipoprotein (HDL) cholesterol, which takes the cholesterol from the rest of the body back to the liver, where it is disposed of. The less LDL and the more HDL cholesterol the smaller the risk of getting clogged arteries. People with diabetes typically have too much LDL and not enough HDL cholesterol, which increases their risk of having a heart attack or stroke.

Cholesterol guidelines for people with diabetes

To help prevent blocked arteries, Diabetes Australia recommends that people with diabetes keep their cholesterol levels within the following ranges:

Total cholesterol	below 4.0 mmol/L
LDL cholesterol ('bad' cholesterol)	below 2.5 mmol/L
HDL cholesterol ('good' cholesterol)	equal to or above 1.0 mmol/L

Foods with a low GI are good for diabetics because the carbohydrates are 'processed' more slowly, so blood glucose levels do not shoot up to unacceptable levels straight after a meal. (Blood glucose sugar levels will rise anyway, and that is why testing should be done two hours after eating a meal to make sure a person's BGL has come back to acceptable levels.) Unhappily potatoes and rice have a high GI rating (but not all varieties of rice—basmati is one with a low GI). Corn has an excellent GI rating and my wife Ros and I have become fond of polenta, which can be mixed with low-fat milk to substitute for mashed potato. Pasta is generally good in the GI department, and you can get very GI friendly varieties if you look for them.

I'm not going to try and deal with the GI issue in great detail in this narrative—there are many excellent books and pamphlets around, complete with great recipes (see 'Suggested reading'). The following Diabetes Australia approved 'Low GI Food Finder' provides a quick ready reckoner, however. Diabetes Australia are keen to encourage as many manufacturers as possible to include the GI symbol and ratings on their products.

Using any of the foods in the list opposite will lower the GI of your diet, and it isn't necessary to eat these foods alone. Eating a low GI food with a high GI food produces an intermediate GI. Pure glucose is rated at 100, and other foods are ranked on a scale from 0 to 100. Low GI foods have a GI of 55 or less.

Eating on the move

Eating the right things at home is much more easily controllable than when you are out or, hardest of all, travelling. Fellow journalist Ross Gittins has adopted the motto: 'Live like a monk at home and don't worry too much when you're out.' Certainly those with Type 2 diabetes have more flexibility than those with Type 1, who must constantly balance what they eat against the insulin they inject. Constant travelling, however, *can* definitely be a health hazard, especially if you live by Ross's maxim.

Now that I have achieved a reasonable control of my BGL, one year on from diagnosis, I'm more relaxed about eating out. You can't expect dinner party hosts to adapt their cooking for the occasional diabetic guest. The answer is to eat moderately, cut the fat off the roast, ignore the cream and take only a few spoonfuls of pudding. Most people will understand when they ask why you haven't scoffed all that has been put in front of you, and you explain.

Q: What is the GI factor?

A: It is a ranking of carbohydrates in food according to their effect on blood glucose levels after eating.

Q: How can I benefit from low GI foods?

A: They cause blood glucose levels to rise more slowly, over a longer period of time than high GI foods, so they help control blood glucose levels.

Q: How should I use the GI factor in my diet?

A: Try to eat at least one serve of low GI carbohydrate foods at each meal, or base at least two meals each day on low GI choices. High GI foods are useful during prolonged physical activity or when treating hypoglycaemia.

Food	*GI Rating*
Biscuits	
Snack Right Fruit Slice	45
Vita-Weat	55
Bread	
Burgen Fruit Loaf	44
Burgen Soy & Linseed Loaf	36
Multigrain 9-grain	43
Cereals	
All-Bran	42
Guardian	37
Porridge	42
Dairy foods	
Custard	43
Ice-cream, low-fat	50
Milk, low-fat, reduced-fat	30
Yoghurt, low-fat, fruit	14–33
Fruit	
Apples	38
Apricots, dried	31
Cherries	22
Grapefruit	25
Oranges	44

Food	*GI Rating*
Fruit (cont.)	
Peaches	42
Pears	38
Legumes	
Beans, baked	48
Beans, soy	18
Chickpeas	33
Lentils	28
Peas, green	48
Pasta and noodles	
Fettucini	32
Macaroni	45
Spaghetti	41
Vermicelli	35
Noodles, instant	47
Vegetables	
Sweet corn	55
Sweet potato	54
Tomato soup, canned	38
Yam	51
Snack foods	
Peanuts	14
Cashews	22

Note: Aim to substitute a high GI food with a low GI food. For example you could change your type of bread or breakfast cereal and eat pasta or legumes more often. Just remember, a healthy balanced diet contains a wide variety of low-fat carbohydrate foods. Courtesy of Diabetes Australia

I began conscientiously enough with airline food, getting myself listed for a diabetic diet. Flying home from an Antarctic voyage, which left from the tip of South America, I had three meals in a row of tasteless steamed fish with corn, enviously eyeing off Ros's chicken in gravy with vegetables, which wouldn't have done me any lasting harm. But I persevered. Flying one day from Melbourne to Sydney I sat next to an architect who noticed I had a special meal. A lettuce sandwich actually.

'Why are you eating that muck?' he asked. I explained I was a Type 2 diabetic.

'So am I. But I'd never list myself as such on an airline. The food is ordinary enough without putting up with the crap they inflict on diabetics.' He said he just ate what he could of the normal meal and got on with it.

Brooding about this I foolishly tried to stay on the straight and narrow and had myself listed on the Qantas computer as a 'white meat vegetarian'—which meant I would have vegetarian meals plus chicken or fish. I didn't fly for about two months, and then waited expectantly for my first 'white meat vegetarian' meal. One of the advantages of 'special' meals is you get served first. I was quite hungry. I opened up my cardboard box (remember the days of hot meals in cattle class?) and found only an apple juice and a forlorn fruit salad comprising chopped up bits of melon. That was it! No bread roll, nothing else. The person beside me had a nice ham, cheese and salad roll, a small cake and even a little packet of macadamia nuts. The cheese would have been a bit naughty, but there was nothing there I couldn't have enjoyed. Well, I would have left the cake, wouldn't I . . .

I asked the flight attendant what had happened to my 'white meat vegetarian' meal. 'Oh', she said, 'all special meals are now fruit'. Just fruit, nothing else. Period. Full stop. That finished me. I'm back on the computer as an ordinary punter. As someone with Type 2 diabetes, I'm more flexible than a Type 1, but surely they would need more than fruit to sustain them between insulin injections when flying! In fact Diabetes Australia recommends people with diabetes take some carbohydrate-laden foods with them—a packet of dried fruit or crackers—when travelling, just in case.

You don't have to be a diet martyr!

Remembering my bewilderment at what I could and should not eat after being diagnosed with Type 2 diabetes, I asked Alan Barclay at Diabetes Australia–NSW, what someone should do under these circumstances:

Alan: I'll tell you what I tell my patients—as well as working with Diabetes Australia I still have a clinical practice and I do still see the newly diagnosed person with Type 2 diabetes—my main focus is on weight reduction. I would usually give people a meal plan that's based essentially on the general dietary guidelines for Australian adults. This means reducing saturated fat, having more wholegrain foods, eating less salt, and not drinking too much alcohol. In other words, general healthy eating. But I try and focus, at first, mostly on cutting the total amount of food people eat.

Tim: Do you look at what they eat and adapt that?

Alan: Absolutely, yes, because it is for life! It is absolutely essential that you first find out people's eating habits but also explore other lifestyle factors. I always ask people whether they work, whether they've got children at home or whether they're married or not, and what their sleeping habits are—so you get an idea of when they're likely to eat and what barriers there will be. For example, if they go on a diet will the kids have a fit or will the husband or wife walk out on them?

Tim: I guess it's terribly helpful if the partner *is* supportive?

Alan: Exactly, particularly for women, because sometimes the male in the family doesn't realise that there's a problem and she might. But it can be the other way around as well. So I always address that psycho-social issue first. Then I get a detailed history of what people are eating now. I feel like the food 'accountant'—I go through in as much detail as possible, amounts as well as the types of food. Then it's essential to try and work around their lifestyle. If I'm advising a businessman who is eating out for two meals a day, there's no point in giving him instructions on what to cook at home. You have to think about what are the best choices in the restaurant or takeaway situation to tailor a diet to the person's lifestyle. Working around the key principles for someone with Type 2 is usually—but not always—weight reduction, so the first step is just reducing the total amount of food people are eating. And not eating between meals. When first diagnosed you don't need snacks. It's a classic mistake people often make when they are first diagnosed. If you're not on medication, you don't need in-between meal snacks. If they do there's a danger they might even start eating more food than they did before! And that won't help with weight reduction.

Tim: This is where the Type 1–Type 2 confusion comes in—people say you must have morning tea and afternoon tea?

Alan: Absolutely unnecessary for someone with Type 2—unless they are on certain diabetic medications. I think three meals a day is very sensible, less of a strain on your pancreas. If you could eat six small meals then that would be fine, but I think what most people do is say I'll have my snacks and I'll have my ordinary meals as well, and they end up eating a bit more food. So I often look at ways around avoiding those sorts of foods, particularly if the person's working. Often the snack foods that are available at work are biscuits or other higher fat foods which are generally not good for diabetes overall. And just generally working diet into the lifestyle, looking at substitutes, I think most people are familiar with that. Having the lower fat alternative to the higher fat one, or at least the lower saturated fat alternative. It's great that as of December 2002 all foods have to have the saturated fats listed on the label. I can proudly say that Diabetes Australia and a few other organisations lobbied the health ministers around Australia hard on that one and we were very happy to get that result as a result of this lobbying.

Tim: Just on that, what should you look out for? I find it all rather confusing. So you look at the saturated fat on a package and what percentage should you try and get below?

Alan: That brings up another issue—what do the figures mean and are there any magic numbers, cut-offs and the like? The figures we generally suggest for fats are based on the Heart Foundation of Australia's recommendations for lipid—that's cholesterol and triglycerides—management. Generally speaking, we'd recommend you look for a food that has ideally less than 10 grams of total fat per 100 grams and, if the food achieves that, then less than 2 grams out of that 10 grams should be saturated. In other words, we're looking at less than 20 per cent of the total fat coming from saturated fat. We've adapted these criteria so they are consistent with the Heart Foundation's recommendations. It also makes it easier for manufacturers and it's consistent for consumers so they know there are not different measures coming out from different health-related organisations.

That works pretty well, 10 grams of fat per 100 grams. It's not the same as the definition of a low-fat food however—it is more generous! By definition low-fat foods have no more than 3 grams of fat per 100 grams. You've probably seen examples of this everywhere, the '97 per cent fat free' type claims. We feel that it is not always necessary to have such low-fat foods. In fact, the ability to make these claims has created a bit of distortion in the food supply, I believe—there are so many of these low-fat foods out there. You may be aware of some of the backlash in the United States against low-fat foods. Often the foods that have become 97 per cent fat free are still as kilojoule or calorie dense as the full-fat products they replaced because they've whacked so much sugar and starch into them—or whatever else they've used to fill it. So there's not a huge reduction in kilojoules when eating them and people often tend to eat them more because they feel that they're so low in fat that they can have an open slather—they think they can eat a whole bucket of this one or that one because it's '97 per cent fat free'. What this has done is increase the population's glycaemic load.

The glycaemic load is the product of the total amount of carbohydrate in a food multiplied by the food's glycaemic index [GI]. One unit of glycaemic load is equivalent to one gram of pure glucose—so obviously your body has to utilise insulin to get rid of that glucose. The higher your diet's glycaemic load, the more insulin your body needs to produce, or you need to inject, to deal with it. Diets with a high glycaemic load have perhaps unsurprisingly been linked to the development of Type 2 diabetes and weight gain. In other words, going for a low-fat food in itself is not necessarily always the best option. Looking for lower kilojoule, lower GI foods *and* the balance of fats is the best way to go.

Tim: The 'poly' and the 'mono'?

Alan: The 'poly' and the 'mono' should be substantially greater than the saturated fat, and if they have made it a lower fat product it's important to look at the kinds of fillers that have been added to it. These can involve starch, sugars, protein or fibre to replace the fat and these may boost the glycaemic load of the food to significantly higher levels. That's where having the GI on the label makes it a lot easier for people because they don't have to try and mentally calculate what impact that's going to have on their blood glucose.

Tim: Are there any 'ready reckoner' information sheets out on how to look at labels?

Alan: Yes, there are a number. Diabetes Australia, Food Standards Australia New Zealand, and many other organisations have resources to help people understand food labels—because it's critical for the empowerment of individuals to help them make informed decisions. The other useful resource Diabetes Australia has is *The Healthy Shopping Guide.* We do a survey every year of one of the bigger supermarkets and we look at every single label of every food in the store, believe it or not. It took us three days last year with three dietitians to do that! A new edition of the book comes out every year. We actually go through with our nutrition criteria and select the foods that are available in Australia for people with diabetes. That's all based on our nutrition criteria, basically on the same principle of no more than 10 per cent fat and no more than 2 per cent saturated fats. We also have criteria for sodium, which addresses the blood pressure side of things—not being too high in salt. For some foods we have dietary fibre and calorie criteria as well, so that they're not too high in calories and, if they're high in carbohydrate, they have a good source of fibre to fill you up.

Tim: That's all pretty involved stuff isn't it?

Alan: It is complicated.

Tim: As a newbie diabetic all I tried to do was to find out the good things to eat and eat them and not think about it too much. Is that too awful?

Alan: No not at all, in fact we surveyed our members back in the year 2000 when the whole label issue was being debated by the food authority and the bottom line was exactly that. Most of our members, like yourself, do read food labels avidly, but when asked if they'd like a simple guide to help them choose food without thinking too hard, nearly 100 per cent said, 'yes, please'. People want to know exactly what is in a food because they want to check nutrition and other claims on the label and they want to have the ability—if it doesn't have a Heart Foundation tick or a GI symbol on it—to be able to make up their own minds. On the other hand, people just want to be able to know that a selected list of foods is fine—it's got a symbol on it, it's in our shopping guide, it's in our handouts and I can trust these foods because Diabetes Australia looks at them every year and you can trust them.

Tim: Can I just pick up on a couple of things? People are obviously going to have to give up some of the foods that they've been eating. I think one of the hardest is dairy products, because that's crammed full of saturated fats—cheeses particularly.

Alan: Dairy products are the number one source of saturated fats in Australia.

Tim: I'd been drinking reduced-fat milk anyway, that wasn't a problem, low-fat yoghurt is fine, a good GI and all the rest of it—but oh dear, no more wonderful cheeses!

Alan: Well, having diabetes does not necessarily mean you will never be allowed to eat your favourite cheese or other tasty morsels again. In fact, there are two schools of thought when it comes to this matter. You may have heard of the 'French paradox'? The French eat a whole range of rich foods, like cheese, and many are high in total and saturated fat, but they do not have the highest rates of overweight or obesity in the world, nor do they have the highest heart disease rates. There are many possible reasons for this but one of the more popular theories is that it is because the French enjoy small portions of their food and make a meal of it and savour it. They also have moderate amounts of red wine throughout the day, and plenty of fruits and vegetables. All these foods are protective against heart disease.

On the other hand, there's what has happened in the United States over the past 20-odd years. They went down the low-fat path and have developed an enormous range of reduced and low-fat foods, and people have been encouraged to eat *more* of them and less of the full-fat alternatives. This is because fat contains twice as many kilojoules per gram as carbohydrates or protein, so the theory is if you eat less fat you will eat less kilojoules and you will lose weight. However, people probably do not enjoy the taste of the lower-fat foods as much, but they think they're doing themselves a favour so they persist. Unfortunately, they may end up eating more food in total, and therefore more kilojoules, so they actually put on weight. Also the more processed lower-fat foods may have less of the protective factors and this is maybe one reason why the Americans get more heart disease then the French.

Anyway, more research is needed on this whole topic.

Tim: I think I'm with the French on that.

Alan: Well at the moment the Australian food industry is certainly pulling us towards the eat more of the low-fat food side. It is possible that this is contributing to the obesity and diabetes epidemic that is gripping Australia at present. But getting back to your original thought, the fat-reduced and low-fat cheeses are very high in sodium—if you've ever looked—double or triple because they've got to give it flavour somehow.

Tim: That's right—otherwise it's like cardboard. What I do—my little treat at lunchtime—is to get good mature cheddar, pull a cheese slicer across for a thin slice, and have it with some honey on a Vita-Weat biscuit.

Alan: Eat it slowly and enjoy!

Tim: Last night we went out for dinner and the usual cheese platter came out. I just had a little bit of each of the blue and the melting brie on a biscuit and just left it at that—it went well with a glass of red.

Alan: As long as you keep this to special occasions I would agree. I don't like people being food martyrs. If someone goes on a diet and gives up every pleasure alarm bells start ringing in my head because it's not sustainable. This has to be for the rest of your life. There are always special occasions. We have a call centre at Diabetes Australia and we get about

500 calls a day in New South Wales. Often the call is from a well meaning relative or friend saying, 'My friend has a birthday coming up, and they have diabetes, what can they eat?' They're looking for some sugar-free, low-fat nightmare that's probably going to taste absolutely foul. I usually say to them, 'Look, it's one time in the year. One meal out of about 1000 or so meals in a year isn't going to kill them. I don't really think it's going to make that much difference. Have a small piece of ordinary cake and enjoy it'. Obviously if you have birthdays for somebody every week then it could become a problem, but if it's your own birthday—and that's what people usually call about—enjoy yourself, have a bit of cake, but make sure it's a thin slice. That way you'll enjoy it more.

Tim: Dare I mention chocolate? It's so awful to consider giving it up. Would, for example, one small square from a block of dark chocolate every day as a treat, be too much?

Alan: Not necessarily. A colleague of ours recently wrote a book about all the wonders of chocolate and certainly it's not as bad as people perceive. Once again it's quantity, and some people can't stop at one square, they have the whole block. What I tend to tell my patients is, 'If you really like your chocolate, buy one of those very expensive little packaged sets where each one's individually wrapped. So you can have one a day and enjoy it, rather than the family blocks where you take one bit, then another and before you know it the whole thing's gone'.

I thought that was really good news on the chocolate front. But it does all come back to self control, which is at the heart of all good diabetic management.

What about high-protein, low-carbohydrate diets?

Dietary fads are constantly feeding—to coin a phrase—the tabloid press, magazines and light-weight—there I go again—television current affairs programs. Debate keeps shifting on the amount of protein that people with diabetes should have in their diet. A high-protein, low-carbohydrate diet contains less than 60 grams of carbohydrate each day—the equivalent of four pieces of fruit, which isn't much. The Dr Atkins diet has less than 20 grams of carbohydrate each day. There have been very few studies that have looked at the effectiveness of high-protein diets for weight loss. Of those few, most have been of relatively short duration—six months.

Those who suffer from diabetes have to consider a wider canvas. It's all very well losing weight quickly—which the high-protein diets do achieve—and then putting it all back on again. Weight loss of any kind improves insulin sensitivity for those with diabetes, which is a good thing. But people with diabetes have to consider the long haul.

Dietitians specialising in diabetes recommend the low-fat, low-sugar diets with a reasonable amount of protein—that is, 12 or 15 per cent of a person's daily energy intake. That could be as little as a 120-gram, palm-sized piece of lean meat. They have reservations about the Atkins style of diet over a long period of time for patients with diabetes.

There can be complications with diets that allow less than 20 grams of carbohydrate a day, which means no bread, no rice and no pasta. This can lead to an increase in dehydration and constipation and a reduction in brain function as well without carbohydrate fuel. There can also be problems with vitamin and mineral deficiencies through lack of cereals, particularly with

Caitlin's fruit cake

This is a personal favourite which my wife Ros makes regularly—great for a morning or afternoon tea snack. Only after you have reached your target weight of course!

Ingredients

1 cup chopped dates
¾ cup sultanas
1 cup milk
1 packet cherries
1–2 grated carrots
1–2 grated zucchinis
1 cup pecan nuts (smashed up a bit)
1 egg
1 cup wheatgerm
1½ cups self-raising flour
1 tablespoon mixed spice
⅓ cup sugar
1 teaspoon bicarb of soda dissolved in a little milk

Method

Pour ½ cup boiling water over dates and sultanas and stand for an hour, then turn once. Then add milk and microwave for 2 minutes on high.

Mix in the remaining ingredients and stir well. It should be very thick and fruity—more ingredients than flour.

Bake in a cake tin or two loaf tins at 180°C for about 1½ hours.

You can put seeds on top if you like.

children. It has been reported that two people who stayed on this kind of low, extreme carbohydrate exclusion diet for six months went temporarily blind because of thiamine deficiency.[2] If you exclude fruit, vegetables and grains—which all have antioxidants, vitamins, minerals and other plant chemicals that do have an association with good health—there is less protection against cancer and heart disease as well.

A long-term low-carbohydrate, high-fat diet is more likely to lead to kidney stones due to the production of more calcium in the urine. People with diabetes have to be very careful about their kidney function. Osteoporosis can also be a problem with a low-carbohydrate diet.

So dietitians dealing with diabetic health recommend the basic principles of balanced, healthy eating—reducing fat intake at first to lose some weight. Just by cutting back on fat and having smaller portion sizes can achieve a four-kilogram weight loss in most people quite quickly. And even that fairly modest achievement is known to have immediate beneficial effects on insulin sensitivity, blood sugar levels and general health.

There are no quick diet fixes for diabetics. It has to be a sustainable diet for life. Lots of vegetables, fruit, wholegrain cereals and low-fat products—and take no notice of media hype about 'miracle' weight-loss diets, celebrity or otherwise. The good news is that there are lots of good, tasty dishes that are diabetically friendly. Don't be a diet martyr!

And remember—we are what we eat.

---

2 Article by Margo Denbe, *American Journal of Cardiology*, July 2001.

CHAPTER SEVEN

Only you can do it

I keep meeting people who are in total denial of their Type 2 diabetes, which I find unbelievable. Take George, an overweight car salesman in his early forties with whom I have had some dealings. I wasn't aware he was diabetic until I mentioned my interest in the condition. He was diagnosed several years ago. So help me God, the following conversation took place:

Tim: So how are you going with your diabetes? How is your BGL?

George: What's that?

Tim: Your blood glucose levels.

George: I wouldn't have a bloody clue.

Tim: Don't you test yourself?

George: I started to, but it was too much of a bore. Frankly I'd rather not know.

Tim: What about your diet then?

George: What diet?

Tim: I don't want to be an alarmist, but if you put your head in the sand you can have nasty side effects down the track.

George: Whatever happens, happens.

Tim: Do you see a doctor at all about your diabetes?

George: Oh yes, I have that three monthly test thing.

Tim: The HbA1c test?

George: If you say so.

Tim: Well that should give you some idea. What is your rating? Is it under 7 or 6 maybe?

George: Dunno—I'm not interested.

Tim: All this will catch up with you eventually, George. Maybe heart attacks, strokes, eye trouble, maybe even kidney failure or amputations. I'm not kidding.

George: I guess I'd rather have a short life and a merry one then.

Tim: The last part isn't going to be fun—not only for you, but whoever has to look after you.

George: So be it.

He then changed the subject.

Assuming that people who read this book do want to take their diabetes seriously, your best friend is you. Essentially this is something individuals have to manage. Without personal motivation, diabetes cannot be controlled. But you do need good information from skilled professionals, which is sometimes hard to come by because the pressure on those professionals is high due to the escalating numbers of people with diabetes.

So who should help you manage your diabetes?

Your first point of contact is probably going to be the doctor who diagnosed you. In my case, Ron was a GP with considerable experience managing the on-going care and treatment of diabetes.

This may not be the case for some people. You should also try and see, as soon as possible after diagnosis, a diabetes team which has a number of members, such as a diabetes educator, a dietitian, and someone to ask advice on an exercise program, which is a vital part of the management of diabetes.

Dr Lilian Jackson is the manager of the Health and Education Division at Diabetes Australia–NSW. She happens to have a medical background as well, but people come to this field from different professions:

Tim: So who are diabetes educators?

Lilian: Most diabetes educators are nurses, but having said that there are some who have a dietitian background or even perhaps a podiatry background. People who are diabetes educators have a background of knowing not only about diabetes, they're also taught education principles. Diabetes educators encourage people with diabetes to manage their own condition. They're taught how to teach, how to get people to set goals and aim towards certain targets and also not to become despondent when things don't always go right—because things don't always go right. Diabetes educators have been shown to be much more effective and much more appreciated by people with diabetes than the medical profession has, in terms of teaching people about how to live with diabetes.

Tim: So after the GP makes the diagnosis how does the contact with a diabetes educator happen?

Lilian: In Australia people are often referred by the GP, but not all GPs will refer you to a diabetes educator. Some people come through Diabetes Australia. We run a diabetes education call centre, where people will ring up and say, 'My doctor told me I had diabetes today', and he may well have told them much, much more, but having heard the diagnosis people very often blank out, they don't hear the rest. Then they go home and the first thought is, 'Oh what am I going to do for food now?' Most people may not know much about diabetes, but they do know it's got something to do with what you eat. So we have a diabetes educator and a dietitian taking calls each working day at Diabetes Australia, but we don't see patients on a one-on-one basis, we refer them—'Where do you live? This is your nearest diabetes centre . . . ring up and make an appointment'.

Tim: Is this referral service something people pay for?

Lilian: No, at the moment it's free. You can ring us up and we tell you where to find the right people. We have a little pamphlet called a locality guide which gives that kind of information.

Tim: Is there any other way to do it?

Lilian: It varies—if you go to a diabetes centre, which can be in a hospital or community health centre. It is usually free, but there are a few private clinics. Some diabetes educators are actually employed by groups of general practitioners or even by endocrinologists—you do not usually pay for that service. The problem is, however, that there are very, very long waiting times for particular diabetes centre-based services and that is really why we instituted our call centre—to assist people in the weeks that they have to wait to get an appointment at a diabetes centre.

Tim: So people just ring up Diabetes Australia?

Lilian: Yes, and we advise them to get an appointment with their local diabetes centre. In the interim period, we send them some information and we invite them to ring if they're in trouble again before they can get to the diabetes centre.

Tim: So how long does this relationship with the diabetes educator continue? I mean first it's, 'Shock, horror, my God, I've got diabetes', then, of course, it's the long haul.

Lilian: You've put your finger on the problem. Theoretically, it should be an ongoing relationship, keeping people up to date with information and education. But there are just not enough resources for that. There are some diabetes centres which do run intermittent up-date groups for people with diabetes. But many can only see the newly diagnosed because they don't have the staff or the time to do more. Being a member of Diabetes Australia is helpful, in that you get a quarterly magazine in each state, and also a national magazine. We run events and seminars frequently and have written resources we can send out to people. Very often, if you attend a hospital diabetes clinic, you may get an up-date seminar arranged by a diabetes centre and, as I mentioned, many divisions of general practice now employ a diabetes educator or a nurse trained in diabetes management. Unfortunately, there are people who fall through the cracks.

Tim: Just getting back to the initial diagnosis—my GP was fairly forthright, which was good for me. He said I had a condition which was not going to get better, and I would have to learn to live with it and control it or I'd be facing very unpleasant side effects. He did say, also, that the diagnosis was a life sentence not a death sentence, and spelt out what I had to do. Does a diabetes educator try and sum up people's different personalities and situations or do they hit them fairly hard?

Lilian: I think that there's one general rule: you don't ever introduce guilt to people. It's not your fault that you have diabetes, even if you weigh 200 kilos. It's still not your fault. There is really, even for all overweight people, a quite considerable genetic background—so you didn't bring it on yourself. Maybe you inherited half the problem, and today's lifestyle is today's lifestyle. It's the way the world operates today. Probably in my grandmother's time they had rolled oats for breakfast because there wasn't cornflakes. We eat processed food, we drive everywhere we have to go. If you're going to the corner shop you drive, you don't walk, even if the shop is only a few metres down the road—it's today's lifestyle. You sit in front of the computer and watch television because the programs are better than they used to be, so it's quite nice watching television. We're all addicted to the news because it's either very good or very bad, but that's the truth of it. Kids are also not eating as healthily as they might and certainly not being as active as they should.

So diabetes educators are not judgemental. They try to educate people to understand their disease, how to cope with it, and with any associated problems that may develop. They also help people to set goals so they can improve their health—but all that can take some time. Of course, they also show people the practical things, how to use their glucometers and monitor their BGL, as well as how to inject insulin using insulin pens, syringes or some of the newer devices, and how to adjust their insulin doses. Diabetes educators also try to make the general public aware of the risk factors for diabetes, not only to themselves but also their families. You can't help it if your family history predisposes you towards diabetes, but some of the risk factors can be minimised through the way you eat and exercise.

Tim: Getting back to policy, as far as possible you give people a pretty realistic assessment?

Lilian: Yes, but as I said, no guilt. We try to encourage people with diabetes to aim for achievable targets. We run events, as I mentioned, to educate groups of people with diabetes and we supply general information on diabetes, the risk factors, information on possible complications, lifestyle strategies, which are important in both the management of diabetes and the prevention of Type 2.

Tim: Of course some people will just be in total denial?

Lilian: Yes they will. But I think there's a lot more awareness and knowledge getting out there now than there was even five or six years ago. Every day in the newspapers there are stories about healthy eating and physical activity. So there is a lot happening now that wasn't happening in the past. But you still can't make everybody do everything. You can give advice, you can give them targets, you can encourage them but we'll never make everybody do everything they should do. One way is to ask them what they would like to do. 'These are the objectives, this is why you should be doing it, these are the ways you could get there—what do you think you could do?'

Tim: But this needs follow up doesn't it?

Lilian: It does really.

Tim: One of the things I found initially depressing was—well it's not cancer, but at the same time, it doesn't get better. There's no cure for diabetes and it will only get worse. Psychologically that weighs on you.

Lilian: Yes, that's true, but today there are many new treatments and management strategies. People can manage many things as long as everybody plays their part and the person with diabetes learns the skills to cope. Diabetes is the first disease where people have had to take charge of it themselves—because you can't take either the diabetes educator or the doctor home with you. You actually have to manage it yourself and I think one of the first steps is to understand that.

You simply have to keep fit

If you were a couch potato before being diagnosed with diabetes—and that may have helped tip you over the edge—it's time to change. Regular exercise is vital for managing diabetes effectively. Walking, cycling, tennis, swimming, it doesn't really matter as long as you do it regularly. Simply walking up stairs instead of taking the lift—helps to get your heart pumping, burning up that pesky glucose.

I have found walking and cycling suits my particular daily routine. But older people sometimes have dicky knees and may find walking painful. That may mean an excursion to the local swimming pool, which usually has a water aerobics program that can be a practical and useful way of exercising—and social too. Even those with arthritis can benefit from limited exercise.

Exercise is all good news. It helps build bone density, increases energy levels, and even reduces stress and anxiety. Apart from making you feel better—by releasing endorphins—it lessens the risks of blood vessel disease, heart attacks and kidney failure, and importantly for those with diabetes, reduces our bodies' resistance to insulin so it can use its own insulin to move glucose from the bloodstream into the cells for energy. So glucose levels drop, cholesterol falls and even blood pressure lowers.

Aerobic is the best exercise, as the heart rate is raised and excess fat is burned off. The trick is to keep doing it every day, or almost every day. This is something your doctor or diabetes educator can advise you about. Some unfit, and admittedly porky, people will have to start slowly and work up to the ideal 30 to 45 minutes or more of exercise each day.

We lose about three per cent of our body muscle mass every year—so if you don't use it you'll lose it—so it is even more important to use your muscles as you get older. Even though you may not lose any weight, fat will be redistributed into muscle—which helps control diabetes. The older you get, the more important exercise becomes to keep your muscle mass up. There are programs for older people which focus on the kind of exercise that keeps muscles strong. It's called resistance training and it may involve doing some work with weights in a gymnasium, and getting an exercise program designed just for you. Or it may be able to be done at home, after consulting your doctor of course!

Some people with diabetes who are on medication or injecting insulin may have to adjust their medication to cope with extra exercise. It is sensible to carry glucose tablets or quick carbohydrate snacks in case your blood glucose levels drop too low during exercise periods. It's also prudent to carry some ID.

The bottom line—and it does have beneficial effects in that department—is that exercise burns up both fats and carbohydrates. Anyway, as they say, just do it!

Talk to a dietitian

It is a good idea to consult a dietitian in addition to a diabetes educator, as soon as possible after diagnosis. I asked Alan Barclay from Diabetes Australia how that could be arranged:

Alan: You can give us a phone call at Diabetes Australia, but we strongly recommend that you see someone personally. In fact, it's a good idea to have your own personal dietitian.

Tim: How often should you consult that person?

Alan: You should try and see a dietitian at least twice in the first year and at least once a year thereafter. I don't think people do see dietitians as much as they should—and that's probably because of lack of access or because of cost. If dietitians were covered by Medicare, it would make a huge difference. (The current Medicare package has helped a bit.) Costs wouldn't be that huge and the savings in the long run would probably be more substantial. But, of course, it often takes five to ten years for those savings to accrue—which is a couple of election terms, sad to say. Basically, the evidence shows that seeing someone to have your questions about what to eat answered gives great benefits. Also it's helpful to have another concerned professional to keep an eye on your weight and body composition. That's something dietitians are particularly good at assessing because it's not just how much you weigh, it's where you carry it. They can try and steer you in the right direction. Nothing beats personalised advice.

Tim: Exactly—and it also motivates people better if they feel that that person actually cares?

Alan: I think dietitians are pretty caring. You tend to spend an hour, at least, roughly an hour on the first consultation, and 15 minutes to half an hour on the follow-ups, which is usually a lot more than you get with your general practitioner.

Going on drugs

As with Type 1 diabetes, Type 2 is with you for life—which is why it has to be managed. Many Type 2 people, like me, are picked up early and can maintain a normal BGL range by losing weight, eating the approved low-fat, low-sugar diet, and exercising. With luck I'll be able to maintain this regime for some years. No-one can predict for how long. Eventually, though, the disease will progress to the point where my valiant pancreas may well still be pumping out insulin, but my body has become so resistant to it that my BGL will begin to rise to unacceptable levels, beyond 6 to 8 mmol/L.

Some people who may have had undiagnosed Type 2 diabetes for many years, may have to commence medication straight away to control their condition. Despite exercise, a conscientious diet and the best of motivation, it will eventually be time for some drug taking. Fortunately, fairly recent research has led to a range of medications being available to keep Type 2 people fit and healthy for many years. There is no shame or disgrace in progressing to drugs—or even insulin injections for that matter—it's all part of the armoury of medical weapons now available to combat diabetes. There are many excellent books available with more detailed information on the different medications for Type 2 diabetes, but I asked Dr Kerry Bowen, an endocrinologist at Royal Newcastle Hospital, to outline the basics:

Tim: Not all people with Type 2 diabetes are overweight are they?

Kerry: That's right—although most people with Type 2 diabetes tend to carry too much weight. To a certain extent Type 2 diabetes may result from a subconscious (or conscious) lifestyle decision. In other words, if you don't exercise enough and if you eat too much, you're more likely to get Type 2 diabetes. If there's a family history of diabetes, that can also be a risk factor. However, if you're not overweight, often medications that make the pancreas work harder are the first choice of your doctor. These medications—and there are different brand names—are known as sulphonylureas. These are usually quite effective in helping to control the blood sugar for a while. They may work for a couple of years, five or even ten years. But eventually they often don't work any more and so you have to have some other treatments when that happens.

Tim: What other medications are available?

Kerry: Well we have the glitazones, which help the body to overcome insulin resistance, but again they're not miracle medications because some people put on a lot of weight when they go on to them, therefore they're not for everybody. They are now available on the Pharmaceutical Benefits Scheme but there are still significant constraints to their prescribing, which means that most of the people who need them won't be able to get them on the PBS. But these medications need to be available for certain people. We certainly don't think that everyone should be on these but there are some people who might benefit significantly from the use of glitazone medication. One group, for example, who have benefited greatly from this medication are truck drivers who might lose their heavy vehicle licence if they were not able to control their diabetes safely without recourse to insulin, and often this medication is the one that saves them from that.

Metformin—some of the brand names are Diabex, Diaformin, Glucohexal—lowers blood sugar by reducing the production of glucose from the liver.

Arcabose is another medication (also known as Glucobay) that can help but it also has some side effects—mainly wind and diarrhoea. But these drugs can sometimes be useful to control BGL. Eventually these tablets will all fail to do the job properly. So you may even be told to go on to one or two, or even three different medications in a recommended combination.

Tim: How do you know when the pills are not working any more?

Kerry: Every three to six months we recommend you have an HbA1c test. This, as you know, is different from measuring your own blood glucose or blood sugar level with a home blood glucose monitor. The HbA1c test requires analysis of your blood in a laboratory and is part of the ongoing management of diabetes. We recommend you have this test done every three months if your diabetes control is not satisfactory, and less often if it's going well. You also know—not only from the test—that things are not going so well if you've got the symptoms of high glucose levels such as thirst, excessive urination, thrush, blurred vision and excessive tiredness. The third way you'll find out if your medication is not doing the job is if your doctor tells you. That's often the case, because you might feel perfectly okay—and that's the trap with diabetes. You feel fine, but your diabetes is not well controlled.

Tim: But why do the pills stop working?

Kerry: Simply because your pancreas won't respond to them any more, it's been flogged and flogged with these pills. Maybe you've gone soft on the sensible eating or the regular exercise, that's a very common reason. Maybe your body's insulin resistance is too strong, or perhaps you're unwell from some other reason unrelated to diabetes. An illness can throw your diabetes out of whack so your diabetes control worsens without you having any good reason for this happening. It's always sensible for you to go and talk to your doctor about that, because there might be something else happening which has made your diabetes more difficult to control. So you might need a check-up to sort these things out.

Tim: So if the pills stop working what should people do?

Kerry: The first call is to your doctor. You may need more diabetes education, from a diabetes educator and a dietitian. Even if you have already seen them after diagnosis, you can forget the lessons learnt. As we know from our school days, lessons need to be repeated until they are learnt, and you may need another session or two. You can also ask yourself if there is anything else that *you* can do to help improve things. That, of course, comes down to the old story of regular physical exercise and sensible eating.

If nothing seems to work any more, it may be time to start on insulin. If this is recommended to you, most likely by your doctor or diabetes nurse educator, then there's not much point in resisting because you've really got to the end of the line when it comes to pills. It's not really worth asking yourself, 'Do I really want to go on to insulin?', because things are not working and you need to move on to something that will work. You might as well accept the inevitable and go ahead and start.

The worst part of going on to insulin is thinking about it. Once you've had the first injection, for most people, it's not a big deal. Many people say that daily finger pricking is more unpleasant than the insulin injections!

Tim: What does insulin do that's so different from the pills?

Kerry: Insulin injections give your pancreas a decent break. If you've got Type 2 diabetes, your pancreas is working overtime to overcome the insulin resistance. That's resistance to your body's *own* insulin. As well, glucose toxicity stops your pancreas from making sufficient insulin; this occurs when the blood glucose level remains high for long periods of time. If you get an injection of insulin, what you're doing is bypassing the need for your pancreas to keep pumping out a lot of insulin. It gives your pancreas a rest and I happen to think that by doing this your pancreas will work better. Your pancreas may not work all that well but it will still keep making *some* insulin and therefore it will help the insulin injections work better as well. You'll smooth out the highs and lows of your blood glucose fluctuations if your pancreas is working a little bit. And, of course, if you've got high blood glucose levels and you're running to the toilet three or four times a night and you're always thirsty and you've got thrush and you feel weak and tired—then by dropping the blood glucose levels those sort of symptoms should go away and you'll feel a lot better.

The other positive thing about switching to insulin is that you will need fewer tablets. I'm not saying that all the tablets will be stopped because there is a good reason to keep metformin going if you're already on that. But some of the other tablets that you may be on for your diabetes will probably be stopped if you switch to insulin. A lot of people tell me they feel a lot better and a lot fitter when they switch to insulin and they sometimes say they should have had done it ten years earlier.

Progressing to insulin can be a bonus

Some people with Type 2 diabetes feel that they have somehow failed in their conscientious control of their disease if they have to progress to medication, and then to insulin injection. This attitude fails to take into account the insidious nature of the disease, which is not only incurable, but affects people in so many different ways. Diet and exercise might control my diabetes—let's say—for the next five years. But someone of a similar age and weight to me might move on to medication after only six months. As Professor Lesley Campbell, Director of the Diabetes Centre at St Vincent's Hospital, Sydney, and a world renowned expert in diabetes research, told me:

> Diabetes is a mean thing. The beta cell—the pancreas—is predestined to run its course through your life. When you get diabetes, the beta cell is already failing. That's why people say, 'One day you'll need tablets', even if you don't. Some people are running out much faster, so basically they need insulin.

Professor Campbell makes the point in her book, *Understanding Diabetes*, that modern insulin therapy is now a far cry from the days when patients had to make up their own injections and then inject themselves with large syringes. Today, disposable plastic syringes with very fine needles that have a special lubricant are available, so that the injection under the skin is barely felt. In fact, most people agree that an insulin injection hurts far less than the pinprick required for BGL tests. In addition, pen devices, which are simple to use and very convenient when you are away from home, are available.

'Most people', Professor Campbell says

> . . . are quite ignorant about modern insulin administration, which is one of the reasons for their fear and reluctance to start treatment. Until fifteen years ago, patients were usually admitted to hospital to start insulin. Nowadays this is rarely necessary. With the help of a specialist diabetes nurse educator, virtually everyone can be stabilised on insulin as an outpatient.

Insulin treatment in people with Type 2 is a little different than for those with Type 1. First, people with Type 2 are older. Second, they are still making and releasing some of their own insulin. Third, very tight control of blood glucose levels may not be absolutely necessary nor even desirable. The type of insulin, the number of injections per day, the method of administration and the dose of insulin will usually be established at the time of initial stabilisation. The insulin regimen may, of course, be changed from time to time if one of the goals is not being satisfactorily achieved.

Professor Campbell says that, occasionally, metformin is prescribed in combination with insulin:

> This is particularly useful in the overweight or in someone who requires very large doses of insulin. This is because

metformin makes the body more sensitive to insulin—whether that insulin is produced by the person or administered by a syringe (or pen device). If the blood glucose control is not adequate when taking tablets and insulin, it usually is best to stop taking the tablets and take the insulin twice daily.

One of the inevitable consequences of insulin therapy is weight gain. Most studies have shown that between two and four kilograms of weight is gained, although one recent study demonstrated an average ten-kilogram weight gain! Some weight gain is largely unavoidable, but it can be limited by an appropriate exercise program and diet, and sometimes by the use of metformin with the insulin. Some weight is regained because the improvement in blood glucose levels prevents continuing loss of glucose in the urine.

This was certainly the experience of a friend of mine, Tony Eames, who was 15 stone (95.25 kilos) when he was diagnosed with Type 2 diabetes in middle age fifteen years ago. He managed to get his weight down to 14 stone (89.8 kg); however, when he progressed to insulin—with some relief, he told me, as it made his diabetes easier to control—his weight shot up to more than 16 stone (100.6 kilos). He had been diagnosed when he went for an insurance medical check-up, 'And came away an un-insurable diabetic!'

Tony wasn't surprised at this development because his late mother and a 'slim athletic' younger brother also had Type 2.

I seem to have my mother's medical profile almost exactly. The difference is that she remained a heavy smoker right to the last—and over a couple of years lost both legs from the knee down. Toes, then ankle, then a foot on one leg, followed by the same progression on the other leg. And in hospital she was still bribing visitors to get her some cigarettes! If you are a diabetic, you mustn't smoke as it doubles the damage.

Several years before Tony went for his insurance medical, he went to his GP and described, what he now knows, were the classic symptoms of Type 2 diabetes. 'I even explained that my poor mother was a double amputee diabetic!' But even that failed to ring any bells. 'He said that I must be overworking—and so I continued untreated for a couple more years. With diabetes now a roaring plague, I can't imagine that ignorance or indifference existing today.'

Tony took his diabetes seriously—and altered his diet and took up 'power strolling', as he puts it, for 45 minutes each day. But bad asthma and a circulation problem in his right leg have limited his daily routine:

> I have always been conscientious about my BGL. In fact, I continue to test my blood sugar three to five times daily. What with that and my four daily insulin injections, I know what Saint Sebastian endured to attain his martyrdom! I feel a right prick many times daily.

His high blood pressure is controlled by medication, but he has suffered other side effects from diabetes, including a progressive loss of sensation in his feet, bleeding in the retina of his left eye—treated with laser surgery—and circulation problems in his right leg. He is also on fairly heavy medication—six Diaformin tablets each day as well as four injections of, 'Fairly hefty quantities of both rapid-acting and slow-acting insulin'.

Today Tony's diabetes is managed, not by his GP, but the diabetes centre of a major Sydney hospital. His only criticism of his otherwise excellent treatment is the reluctance of his earlier advisers to move him to insulin when it was obvious—to him—that his regime of medication, diet and exercise wasn't working:

> As you can gather, my form of Type 2 diabetes is particularly bad. It got progressively worse and I've been an insulin junkie now for about eight years. To be honest, I couldn't wait to get on to it because it gave me a grip on a condition that was spinning out of control and undoing my life. My four shots a day have become routine and really quite painless.
>
> I recall once flying into Singapore's Changi Airport after having stupidly left my needle and gear in an inaccessible bag. By then pretty sugared up, I popped into the gents and was steadying the needle ready to stab myself when an American middle-aged man opened the door.
>
> 'Jesus, man! They hang you for that here', he whispered in alarm.
>
> 'Well, if you're hanging out as badly as I am right now, you just take the risk', I replied, holding the needle up towards him. 'Fancy a taste?'
>
> The poor man shot out, quite forgetting whatever had brought him to the lavatory in the first place.

Tony Eames is up-beat about his future, and mine. He was kind enough to write to me not long after my own diagnosis to say that he believed I could keep the lid on my diabetes for years to come. 'I know many Type 2 folks who will never end up on the needle.'

CHAPTER EIGHT

Don't panic!

I didn't ask to join the late onset Type 2 diabetes club, but I found I was a member anyway. I began my membership with the usual mix of ignorance, fear and dread. Was this to be the end of my way of life as I knew it? Untamed high blood sugars threatening to rob me of my sight and my sex life, and also with heart attacks, strokes, kidney failure and possibly amputations—starting with my toes and working upwards.

A joyless—and relentlessly sober—regime of high-fibre vegetables, fruit, fish, lean meat and enough lentils to enable me to fart my way to the diabetes clinic without using the car? I mean one of the compensations of growing old is that the enjoyment of good food and wine seems to appreciate rather than diminish—unlike some other inevitably fading physical functions. Of course it wasn't as bad as all that, as I hope I've been able to make clear in the course of this narrative.

Alcohol—admittedly in distressingly small amounts—has a beneficial effect on the health of Type 2s and everyone else—didn't we always know! And sugar isn't the bogey it was once thought to be. It's just another carbohydrate, and we need that to function properly. So the occasional chocolate or honey on toast isn't going to nudge us noticeably closer to that final rendezvous with the undertaker. And there are mercifully all manner of diabetes-friendly and agreeable foods to delight the palate, when you look into it.

As I battled to cope with finger pricking, blood glucose readings, HbA1c tests, a modified diet—and smaller portion sizes—the arcane mysteries of the glycaemic index and the appalling consequences of saturated fats, I became aware that many people I knew were also members of the Type 2 club. This had escaped my notice until I joined too. Some were models of rectitude—but perhaps that is an overstatement. Others were distressingly cavalier, like my acquaintance George mentioned previously, who was in total denial. I was interested to talk to some of them about their tussles with Type 2—and share their experiences.

Ross Gittins

Ross is the Economics Editor of the *Sydney Morning Herald*, and we share the common bond of journalism as well as Type 2. I wasn't aware that Ross had diabetes until a mutual friend told me. He was diagnosed by his family doctor at the age of 47, when he needed a medical examination for insurance and superannuation purposes:

My quack took one look at me, decided I looked like a prime suspect for diabetes. He whipped out his little blood testing kit, told me to stick out my finger while he pricked it, and soon pushed over to me the little calculator thing showing my BGL was 15 [mmol/L].

'There you are', he said. 'You're a diabetic.'

In all my subsequent visits I've been paying him what amounts to a spotter's fee. (I'm very grateful to him, though I'd never admit it to his face.)

Although Ross didn't know it at the time, his father's side of the family was 'riddled' with diabetes. His sister had Type 2 and her daughter Type 1, as well as a cluster of diabetic uncles. Like me, he knew nothing about diabetes. 'My motto was never trouble illness, 'til illness troubles you.' He was diagnosed shortly before he was due to take his family on a hiking holiday through the Lake St Clair–Cradle Mountain National Park in Tasmania, a six-day guided walk. He was keen to do that, so he took to the streets of Glebe, marching about with a hiking pack laden with roof tiles!

I love bushwalking and intended to do it a lot when I retired (I had resolved several years earlier that I wanted to do every major walk in the South Island of New Zealand before I croaked). However, I'd been putting on weight and I started to fear that, by the time I was able to devote a lot of time to walking, I'd be too unfit to do it. The diabetes thing was forcing me to get fit and stay fit and so I regarded it as a blessing in disguise.

Ross's diagnosis coincided with his then 16-year-old daughter turning vegetarian, so the whole family decided to join her—

with occasional meat eating lapses in her absence or at restaurants. On the advice of his GP, Ross went to the diabetes centre at Royal Prince Alfred Hospital to have his diagnosis confirmed:

> They gave me a lot of good literature and sent me to Diabetes Australia to join up and get more books and equipment. I studied it up with great interest—and became a menace to my friends spouting on about it. To this day I try to keep up to date by reading Diabetes Australia's quarterly *Conquest* magazine from cover to cover—not an onerous task.

He says he was never depressed by being diagnosed with Type 2, nor has he been since. When he lost weight—since put back on—his wife decided getting diabetes was the best thing that had happened to him. Ross didn't disagree. 'Her point was that without becoming a diabetic I would have just got fatter and more unfit until I carked it at an early age.'

Fast walking in his suburban streets became his main exercise, for 35 to 40 minutes four times a week:

> I started going to the Sydney Uni Women's Sports Union gym (they made me an honorary woman) once, then twice a week. In the last year or so I've acquired a personal trainer who, for an exorbitant fee, absolutely knackers me once a week and requires me to go another two times a week, to knacker myself yet again.
>
> For someone who never played sport as a kid and had never exercised, I've had surprisingly little trouble maintaining my exercise regime regularly since 1995. As a columnist who writes on certain days, I have a very predictable, regimented week. I've simply built my exercise sessions around my column days and I stick to it. My doc says I've become addicted to the

release of endorphins and I think he's probably right. Exercise has become my one main hobby. I totter away from sessions with my trainer—he pushes me just up to the limit of what I can take—but I actually look forward to being done over by him.

Ross Gittins has had diabetes now for eight years, and until two years ago, controlled it with diet and the aforementioned mildly addictive exercise. He is now on medication. He admits to still carrying too much weight, now about 100 kilos, after getting down to the 90s. (He was around 107 kilos when diagnosed.) He has no problem acknowledging that he has diabetes—as will be evident from this contribution—but doesn't necessarily tell everyone he meets. 'To me, it's old news'. So far he has not suffered any discrimination as a person with diabetes, but has read enough about that issue in *Conquest* to realise that it is a problem for some.

He has managed to keep the complications of diabetes at bay, with no problems yet with his eyes, feet or kidneys. But three years ago he began suffering angina attacks, and had a quintuple heart bypass—which was completely successful:

Tim: Has having diabetes made you more or less optimistic about the future?

Ross: I think whether you're optimistic or pessimistic about the future has more to do with your general personality and outlook on life than with diabetes as such. I very early reconciled myself to the likelihood that I'll live a shorter life than a lot of people. What of it? Overweight and unfitness would probably have carried me off early anyway. In any case, out of sheer selfishness I'd want to die before my wife did—diabetes or no.

Tim: What would your advice be to someone newly diagnosed with Type 2 diabetes?

Ross: It's your life and your body—take responsibility for managing your own condition. Doctors are just people I pay to give me expert advice in the management of my body. I invariably take their advice—but not before I've sought to understand it and put them through their paces. (And every decent doctor prefers to have patients who take such an attitude.) Apart from that—get over it! Diabetes Australia's *Conquest* is excellent for its unending stream of real life stories of people achieving great things with their lives despite their diabetes. After the initial adjustment phase, you're only entitled to feel sorry for yourself if you have a real lot of trouble establishing good control.

Moira Rayner

Moira is a well known—and feisty—lawyer at the forefront of policy development, not only in Australia but overseas as well. Her jobs have ranged from Chairman of the Western Australian Law Commission in the early 1990s, to Victoria's Commissioner for Equal Opportunity. Somehow she finds time to be a journalist and author, and take unusual overseas gigs, as she did in 2000 when she went to London to establish the Office of Children's Rights Commissioner in London. When I contacted her to ask about her experiences with diabetes, she was a member of Western Australia's Anti-Corruption Commission.

Moira was 48 when she was diagnosed with Type 2, and for someone who has specialised in discrimination, perhaps she was well positioned to have a bad experience:

Moira: I had been feeling very unwell—tired, cantankerous, failing eyesight for quite some time—and seeing a GP quite often, who assured me there was no physical cause and maybe I had chronic fatigue syndrome. This was not helpful. I had a prolonged time of general unwellness while in Scotland for a few weeks, I couldn't understand why I couldn't read the street signs and felt so exhausted and had a few symptoms such as boils and thrush. Then I had a very bad fall while on holidays which caused extensive, deep bruising and shock—that was the second time I noticed that my eyesight had become blurred. I went on with my holiday. Later I realised that I had had a deep vein thrombosis and I was a very lucky woman not to have killed myself, because I didn't seek medical attention for the swollen leg and chest pains. Oh dear.

However, a few weeks later I slipped and hurt my ankle and saw my GP, who assured me it was a sprain. I continued to feel worse generally in my health and made complaints—I had started losing a lot of weight, which she thought was good! I was also peeing constantly, had an insatiable thirst, really couldn't read at all, had bad thrush and a couple of delicate and painful boils, and felt confused, exhausted and extremely bad-tempered. My GP could only suggest I take more time off and see an optometrist about my vision.

By this stage I realised we had a communication problem. So I got an X-ray myself through my physiotherapist and took the evidence of a fracture into my GP, and said firmly: 'Look, I've got diabetes. I know I've got diabetes. Please organise the blood tests.' I was assured that I didn't have diabetes. The next morning when the results were in the GP rang and said I was right, and I should see a specialist and, 'Watch my carbohydrates'. Very helpful.

Tim: Did you have any history of diabetes in your family, and did you know anything about the disease?

Moira: My grandfather had diabetes, which was a huge family issue. I did not know the difference between Type 1 and Type 2 diabetes, however. He lived on a very limited diet—lean meat, an ounce of cheese a day, plain vegetables and cups of milky tea, no desserts or fruit. He was very constipated and actually died of bowel cancer, so there's a lesson in that. He had perfectly good eyesight and no other complications of the disease and normal BGL all the time. He never took any medication for his diabetes. We all knew he couldn't eat sugar or cakes or lollies, that he had to watch his feet and wear soft shoes.

I knew what the symptoms were from general reading, but nobody ever suggested I was likely to inherit it. In fact none of his children, my mother included, ever got tested for it—until she had an accident in her eighties, and was found to be diabetic as well—a strange oversight. I knew, because a family friend had gone blind and later died of complications, that diabetes was a serious illness and that it could be managed by diet and exercise in some cases.

Tim: How did you react when you found out you had Type 2 diabetes?

Moira: I was pretty upset but also relieved because I knew that I could do something about it and that I wasn't going mad. I set out to learn everything about it and changed my diet and other habits overnight. My greatest fear was of going blind. I was so relieved to find that my eyesight would return!

As I started to feel so much better, I realised how ill I had been feeling for so long. It was like a dark cloud lifting.

I knew it couldn't be cured and it was up to me to manage it. I was determined not to go under, and not to go on medication and not to get any complications. I did not believe my specialist who said I would get complications, and I still don't believe it. I started doing a lot of work on my health, which mostly involved keeping a close eye on my BGLs with a meter and keeping a diary. I also joined a field test, run by St Vincent's Hospital, of a drug to reduce blood cholesterol, the side effect of which is regular check-ups of cardiac, blood sugar, cholesterol and vision health, which I have found enormously helpful. I see them at least twice a year.

Tim: Can you remember what your blood glucose levels were when you were diagnosed?

Moira: Between 25 and 30 mmol/L, as I recall. Very high!

Tim: How was your state of mind when you were eventually diagnosed?

Moira: I was already depressed because I was feeling so dreadful. I was relieved, and invigorated. It prompted me to change not only my lifestyle but also my working arrangements and career. I even joined a gym! In fact I got my blood glucose levels back to normal levels in three months, which I thought was bloody good.

For the first four months I couldn't do much because I was on crutches, but that was exercise too! I made sure I got at least 40 minutes walking a day. I find daily exercise essential to keep blood sugars within limits. It also makes me feel a great deal better.

Tim: Do you keep taking your BGLs?

Moira: I kept it up for many years. In the last couple of years this has dropped off a bit, which is a big mistake and I allowed my weight to creep back up, which required me to go on to medication [Metformin], which I am working on to ensure it will be temporary. I try to take my BGL each morning and whenever I'm feeling unwell, and on a variety of occasions during each day, just to keep in control. I have to take at least 20 minutes moderate exercise a day. Six small meals. In the last couple of years I have given in to a tendency to resent the diet restrictions and to sneak a sweet thing and try to cheat. Fool! That's how my friend—whose diabetes is no worse than mine—ended up on insulin.

Tim: What was your weight when you were diagnosed, and did you succeed in reducing it?

Moira: I was about 98 kilos. I dropped 25 kilos in four months. I have since slipped up and put on another 7 kilos and have to keep working on it.

Tim: What about alcohol? Did you cut down and have alcohol-free days each week as recommended?

Moira: Don't be silly! I had a very wise specialist who recommended keeping it to two glasses of a really good red. It helped. It helps.

Tim: Do you tell people you have diabetes when you travel, or go out?

Moira: I take sugar-free gum with me, and stick to fruit for dessert. I don't tell people I'm diabetic—I tell them I'm a vegan, which is true, and is much more disturbing and difficult to cater for, so you can't be too picky. I get vegan food on airlines, and when I am at a person's home for a meal I eat around what's offered, otherwise you become precious and a bloody nuisance and anti-social. I will tell people I have diabetes when they try to insist on my having a chocolate or something that will clearly make me feel really crook, and it shuts them up.

Tim: Political correctness recently decreed that a person with diabetes should not be called 'a diabetic' but instead, a person with diabetes. What do you think about that? Are you unhappy about being labelled as 'a diabetic'?

Moira: It is not political correctness. I am not my condition. I am a middle-aged lawyer with a penchant for speaking out on unpopular issues who happens to have a number of 'conditions' including post menopausal hot flushes, middle-aged eyesight, firm opinions and a desire to change the world. I don't like limiting labels much. I say, when I do, that 'I am diabetic' not 'I am *a* diabetic', so I suppose the PC concept is better. Interestingly, in the United Kingdom the preferred label is 'disabled people' not people with disabilities, so political correctness varies according to the locale.

Tim: After living with diabetes for some years how has your attitude to the disease changed with time? Are you more optimistic about the future than you were, or pessimistic?

Moira: As optimistic as when I started, though I expect to have a shorter life. This means I will only make it to 91 instead of living to 106 as my great grandfather did. Diabetes does not dominate my life. It is not a cause of sadness, but irritation, especially when it comes to not eating gorgeous desserts, and I am sad that I have had to cut out cheese, which I love and know quite a bit about. It's one of the reasons I became a vegan.

Tim: What would you say to a person recently diagnosed with Type 2?

Moira: It's a great opportunity to grab a fresh hold on your life and make decisions about living a healthier and happier one. I wish I had known years earlier—I would not have been so damned difficult to live and work with, and would have had to make a lot fewer apologies for crabby reactions and occasional confused thinking. Some would say more than occasional confused thinking. Get out into the fresh air, do as much walking as you can and, if you can, get into weight lifting—it does wonders. Normalise the new ways of eating, exercising and managing your life and its pressures, which are actually perfectly normal, healthy choices. Nobody needs to know it's special for you.

I don't feel apologetic about taking more rest, for example, than I used to, or making choices about not taking on unnecessary work stress—which does affect BGL substantially. You can manage diabetes—a friend of mine has effectively become non-diabetic—a lot easier without medication by simply adopting a healthier lifestyle. Don't think of yourself as sick, just someone who needs to be a bit more careful about your health.

Over the last four months I got really fed up with being constantly rather 'high' on the BGL and feeling crook. So I bit the bullet and really got into the gym work—though I am still overweight, and nobody better get on my case about that, because that's what I am, though it is coming off—working with a personal trainer twice a week, doing boxing (yes, real stuff with gloves and bags and things) and other very vigorous exercise, including weights up to five days a week. It's making me feel quite marvellous. I would never have done this if I hadn't got a disease that could turn me into a cripple if I let it.

Tim: What about the 'guilt' syndrome?

Moira: I get pissed off with people who assume that Type 2 is a disease that you brought upon yourself by being overweight or self-indulgent and inactive. This 'blame' is peddled by the medical profession. I was not inactive—for many years I walked vigorously for at least 45 minutes a day. Yes, I've always been overweight, but 'fat' is something that everyone seizes on and blames you for. This is a great disincentive to doing anything about it.

If I had been told of the particular risk to me because of the family connection and the precise need to take preventive measures I would have taken it seriously. The level of public ignorance is vast—a trained nurse seriously told me that it's because I 'ate too much sugar', which was never the case. I get quite stroppy with strangers who tell people with diabetes that they are lazy and who have the nerve to be disapproving if, in their uninformed opinion, you 'shouldn't' eat something that has a little sugar in it. Fat in food is much more significant as you know.

Peter Bower

I've known Peter for quite a long time. When we lived in Sydney we had sons the same age, now well and truly grown up. As coincidence would have it, Peter lives in the same 'sea change' area as I do on the mid north coast of NSW, where he is an education administrator. I hadn't registered that he had Type 2 diabetes until I signed on myself.

Peter, as they say, is a good 'tooth' man—very fond of his tucker. A year ago we met for lunch at a local poker machine palace. He found one, very generous I thought, main course not enough so he lined up for a second, as well as a substantial dessert. I remembered this—and realise belatedly that he must have had diabetes then. To this day he carries a generous paunch, not recommended for a member of the Type 2 diabetic club. Peter was diagnosed about ten years ago during a check-up he decided to have when was approaching 50. He was fine—except that his doctor told him he had late onset diabetes. He must have had Type 2 for a while, because he went straight on to medication. To this day, Peter doesn't test his BGL regularly—in fact he doesn't even have a glucometer. He relies on his three monthly HbA1c test to chart his progress, but is uncertain about his status:

Tim: Did having diabetes change your life in any way?

Peter: I think I was more conscious of my weight then. I think I might have modified my diet and had less cakes and pastries and that sort of stuff, but I didn't do a 180-degree turn.

Tim: Did you go to any diabetes health meetings?

Peter: Yes I did. I went to Royal North Shore Hospital for a session on how to diet. I was very pleased about that, because I told them what I ate and how often I ate, and the dietitian at the time said, 'You've got no worries. You are eating everything that you should be eating without me changing your diet. In fact don't change a thing.' She even said at that stage, 'You can eat as much as you like'!

Tim: Did they make you aware of the dangers of saturated fats and that kind of thing—dairy products and cheese?

Peter: They made me aware of that, but apart from meat, I don't have a lot of that stuff at all.

Tim: You are carrying too much weight, like most of us do. Did anyone suggest you took that off?

Peter: Yeah, absolutely.

Tim: Did you do anything about it?

Peter: I thought about it and I tried to, but exercise for the sake of it bores me. I started walking. When I came up here I started walking up and down the beach, walk, walk, walk and it was boring. I even bought an exercise bike, but I have a problem with sitting on a bike for all that time. My aim was to sit in front of the TV after dinner and ride the bike, but that didn't work. So the bike had to go. But since I've been up here, the guy next door is very active, he is my age, and I have a new table tennis table and we play table tennis as much as we can for over an hour. I put a heavy top on, and the perspiration streams out of me and I love it.

Tim: What about your diabetes care up here? You are in diabetic heartland! What approach did your new GP take when you arrived?

Peter: Just keep taking the Diabex, watch your diet, and he sent me along to the diabetes health service. I went to one of those meetings on how to lose weight. Look, I must tell you about losing weight and what my theories are. I believe food is a minor contributor to weight gain and obesity. The biggest contributor to weight gain and obesity in our civilisation is the fact that our jobs and work are becoming more and more sedentary. Many truckies have weight problems. In the white collar area I have seen people who were as fit as buck rats who used to teach in schools, which means they walk around all day long, pointing up to the board, carrying things around, they are like normal people.

And they come in here to a desk job and within a few months you can't recognise them. They are like battery hens.

Tim: Sure, that's a recognised factor that sedentary jobs contribute. But it's also a known thing about Type 2 diabetes that carrying too much weight is not a help.

Peter: It can be a chicken and egg thing. In my view it's questionable which comes first, diabetes or the obesity.

Tim: I've seen you double up on main courses. To be blunt, isn't that suicidal behaviour for someone with diabetes?

Peter: If I go out, I say to hell with it, I'm going to indulge myself.

Tim: What about grog?

Peter: I am vigilant about what I drink. It's parsimonious and I do have alcohol-free days. But I'll have a few drinks if I go out, or if people come over and I am in a position to go for it without driving.

Peter told me he has not yet had his feet checked by a podiatrist, but does have regular eye checks because he has poor eyesight in any case. I was concerned that he was not testing himself for blood glucose, and that he seemed unaware of his exact status, even with his three-monthly HbA1c tests:

Tim: Peter, would it be fair to say that diabetes sits pretty lightly on your shoulders? Take the pills, do certain things that you know you should do, like exercise and eating vegetables . . .

Peter: That's correct. I try to go along with it, but I don't let it rule my life. While my tests are okay, not deteriorating, and my local doctor keeps on saying to me, 'You are doing all the right things, your tests are the same . . . '

Tim: But with respect, you *aren't* doing all the right things. There is an argument that you should be proactive in this.

This is something that doesn't get better, it only gets worse. Diabetes is a chronic condition. It can overtake you in later life in all kinds of terrible ways—strokes, heart attacks and that's not the half of it. I'm suggesting to you that perhaps you ought to be doing more to help yourself...

Peter: I'm quite sure what you say is right. But I look at it this way—I believe that doctors shouldn't run our lives. Health is such enormous industry. A few decades ago I would have been considered a pretty fit 63-year-old and given the three score years and ten target—Christ I look like getting there. But now people talk about greater longevity, and there's a whole industry out there. I am a bit of a cynic about a lot of this.

Okay, you say diabetes sits lightly on me. But I've got to 63, I'm still reasonably okay for my age, so I don't want to get worried about everything.

Tim: All that is fine, except that the big flaw is weight.

Peter: I've lost weight, particularly with table tennis. I'm conscious of the fact I should be weighing less. I'm eating as well as I can. In the morning I have two Weetbix, I have some sultanas, I have a banana and I have milk on it and a cup of tea—and psyllium husks and orange juice. Lunch is a sandwich and fruit. For dinner I eat too much. That is one meal when I am not parsimonious. Cauliflower, broccoli, veggies and meat.

Tim: I'm told it's not the best meal of the day to have as a big one, but we all do!

Peter: I like the effect of a large meal. A bit like alcohol, it is relaxing. If you have a nice big meal and you are working, it is relaxing. Your body digests it and you let down. At night I find it pleasant. Remember that my first diet counsellor at

North Shore said, 'You can eat as much as you like. That's a very reasonable diet'.

Tim: With respect I'd query that! Going by what I've been told that doesn't sound good advice.

Peter: I don't think that is good advice either. It's a bit like saying to an alcoholic you can have two or three bottles of wine a night and don't worry!

Tim: Are you optimistic about your diabetes?

Peter: I'm accepting.

Tim: Do you think you will live until you are 80?

Peter: I don't care! Quite frankly, if I don't have a good quality of life, or a reasonable quality of life . . . I'm not a cricketer wanting to get the magic ton or whatever. I've had a good life. I've quite enjoyed it, and while ever my mind and my body is okay . . . My big fear is that something will happen to me and I will be out of control, that I won't be able to make decisions for myself. I'm not a religious person, and I believe that there is no-one up there—or down there—waiting for me, and I believe intellectually in euthanasia. I don't feel I've got a lot to look forward to, or that life has a helluva lot to offer me that I haven't already seen or experienced.

The older I get, in many respects, the worse off my quality of life is going to be. No-one is saying, 'As you get older there are all these good things that are going to happen to you'. There are not good things that are waiting to happen. Socially—in fact in every way—the older you get, the less you are living life to the full. So I've got to the stage where I ask what more is there that life is going to offer me, that I'm really hanging out for? And I can honestly say I can't think of a lot. So as long as my quality of life is reasonable,

I'll hang in there. But I'm not worried about a sort of chronological benchmark, like 80, 90, 100 or 120.

Tim: A good quality of life as long as you can have it?

Peter: Yes.

Eva Cox

When I asked Eva how she wanted to be described in the context of this book she wrote, 'Academic, shit stirrer and commentator'. So I thought it best to flesh this out a bit, and trawled the internet for her CV. It turns out she is one year younger than I am, both born before World War II, but we could not have entered the world under more different circumstances. Eva Hauser was born in Vienna and soon declared non-human and stateless by Hitler, growing up as a refugee in England until 1946, then in Rome until 1948 and arriving in Australia at the age of ten. I grew up in peaceful Tasmania, but was not unaffected by the war because my father joined the AIF and went to the Middle East—and fortunately returned.

With such a background it is hardly surprising that Eva is committed to social policies and the rejection of injustices. She has become one of Australia's best known—and forthright—commentators on politics and society. She was selected to present the ABC's Boyer Lectures in 1995, titled *A Truly Civil Society*.

We met, unexpectedly, at the Sydney Writers' Festival in 2003. To be honest I didn't recognise her at first. She seemed to have halved in size. Type 2 diabetes provided the weight-loss incentive, of course. Like me she was diagnosed in her early sixties, and another parallel was that we were both picked up in a routine medical check without any symptoms whatsoever—other than high blood pressure:

Tim: How did you react to the diagnosis at first?

Eva: Scared! A friend had died recently, so it frightened me as she had ignored her diabetes and had a heart attack. I then decided to take control by finding out what I could.

Tim: Were you surprised to find how many of your friends had diabetes once you realised you had it yourself? And did you talk to them about how they managed their diabetes and draw any comfort or motivation from them?

Eva: No, because others are not keen to talk about it as it's a dag's disease, so a few tried to act as though they didn't have it. I didn't find diabetes part of a shared/sharing supportive community and I think that reflects the wider society. Why are people so reluctant to talk about it? They often bore you shitless with other allergies and problems regarding food and so on.

Tim: May I ask how much weight you actually lost?

Eva: As I said on Robyn Williams's *Science Show* on Radio National, I was once a 110 kilo plus weakling. I am now a trim 70 or so kilos. This process took just over a year, with the bulk literally disappearing over eight months and stabilising for the same time. Losing this amount of weight's been very good for me in many ways as I am more energetic, less anxious, more comfortable with myself and enjoy buying clothes again.

Tim: How did you do it?

Eva: Not in any recommended way! I didn't go to a nutritionist or follow any particular specified diet plan and I can't tell you exactly how much I lost because I didn't even weigh myself before trying to control my leaping blood sugar. I started exercising, but didn't play sport, go to a gym or hire a personal trainer. I did not join a weight watch program or even join a group. I started walking more but still don't like it much as I have flat feet, so I only walked when I was going somewhere close by, rather than driving.

Tim: Was it hard to find out what you could eat?

Eva: I read a lot about diet and diabetes, discovered low and high glycaemic foods and thought this made sense. I was very good at pigging out on comfort food and had noted that mash, white bread and rice seemed to become very 'more-ish' as did sweet stuff. So I thought I'd try to exclude those and that meant I ate less. I also just cut down on other foods, such as fats, which were high in calories.

Tim: Most people who diet start off with good intentions and then fall by the wayside.

Eva: How I did it was important. I am very good at undermining any virtuous goals I set myself, so I drifted into managing my food intake in ways which were not very demanding. I realised setting firm and disciplined criteria for eating gave me infinite possibilities of transgressing and failure, so I adopted something I'd read about and tried before. I didn't give anything up, I just decided not to eat it at that time. I remembered that was how I gave up smoking. I make a point of finding flavour in small morsels, such as olives, and basically indulged via small tastes rather than satiation. I'm a keen cook and foodie, so it's quite hard.

Tim: What about exercise?

Eva: I work out for half an hour daily to Radio National's *AM*, reading the paper while working with ankle weights to the duller bits, then listening while using the dumbbells to more interesting items. I discovered early morning endorphins were energising, but as I had less to carry it became easier too. So now I seem to have stabilised, with normal blood sugar readings and lots of clothes I like and not just fat lady gear.

Tim: What irritates you about having diabetes?

Eva: The culture of 'blame'. That somehow people with diabetes 'brought it on themselves'. Fat busters of the world unite! You are becoming scarily fashionable as we are constantly told the new epidemic is obesity. The media produce daily stories on how sloth and overeating will cost us dearly in the long run. Fat is becoming the new symbol of sin, the sign of antisocial and irresponsible self indulgence. Gym junkies have, for some time, made their exercise addiction a personal and social virtue, but now food is being allied with sloth. The obese person becomes the new symbolic sinner, irresponsibly behaving in ways which will result in increasing health costs and burdening taxpayers. I can't bear those who say smugly that I caused my diabetes by being overweight, ignoring the many overweight people who are not diabetic and the people with diabetes who are thin.

This ploy of many health promotion messages assumes that a mix of information and willpower can fix what are called lifestyle diseases. This ignores the evidence that there are many, many causes of obesity, both physical and social, and assuming we want to be fat is not helpful. So I'm not going to claim that anyone can do it by just will and self control. I didn't and am not sure what worked for me but there were some coinciding stimuli, ranging from fear to a recognition of the personal and social factors that made me use food for comfort and a greater understanding of how my body treated food.

Tim: So what can be done about these 'fattist' attitudes?

Eva: The first thing is for the policy makers and our families and so called friends to stop making us feel bad about ourselves. As fat people, it only makes many of us crave more food. I realise that I often ate to manage anxiety and feeling bad. The second is for the manufacturers and fast-food groups to stop inundating us with messages that their snack foods, high in crap, are the way to happiness and social acceptance. So stop making overweight people feel guilty, as it doesn't work for most of us.

Tim: How do you feel about your future now?

Eva: I've had a few collywobbles and moments of severe doubt, particularly when reading about the general prognosis of diabetes. I know that scaring people can work but it can also induce a feeling of hopelessness. So along with not blaming us for our purported sins that made us diabetic, maybe the pundits need also to recognise that too much gloom and doom may make it hard to be 'good'. I am now quietly optimistic, mostly because I keep my levels stable and normal with low levels of medication, diet and exercise. So far so good, there are no adverse signs apart from a small change in glasses prescriptions.

Tim: What are your expectations?

Eva: I hope a long and healthy life but I know statistically that is less likely now than before. Will diabetes get me, will I suffer some serious disabilities? I am still in full-time paid work, despite being what a friend calls the statutory age of senility (65). I feel that continued contact with students is useful and I intend to continue that. I feel at my age my contribution is to be outrageous, to push boundaries younger women can't because of career issues. So I will continue to do so and I hope to remain healthy while doing it.

CHAPTER NINE

Looking ahead

So am I a diabetic or not?

I ask this rhetorical question not because I am in any doubt that I have Type 2 diabetes, but whether I can describe myself as 'a diabetic'. Political correctness says not, I am 'a person with diabetes'. Personally, I have no problem declaring 'I am a diabctic'. To me, it's rather like saying 'I am a journalist', rather than 'A person with journalism'. (Some would equate that profession with an incurable, vexatious condition.) It was not until I had begun research for this book that I became aware of this semantic sensitivity, and asked many of the people I interviewed whether they objected to being described as 'A diabetic'. Most didn't, and some did.

Moira Rayner said that she was 'not her condition', and preferred to say 'I am diabetic' rather than 'I am *a* diabetic'. Eva Cox, on the other hand, who is no friend of discrimination in any shape or form, says bluntly that she finds this particular issue 'A crappy argument' and she hates the use of PC in this way. Crime writer and Type 1 diabetic Peter Corris was dismissive of such PC, and fellow journalist Ross Gittins thinks it is simply silly. Contributor Tony Eames was even more blunt:

> A person with diabetes is a diabetic. I have diabetes, ergo I am a diabetic! What are those fools doing with our language? Is a choleric individual now to be referred to as, 'A person with cholera'?

Yet, as I was to discover quite quickly, this is an issue regarded seriously by health professionals, particularly by Diabetes Australia. I raised it with Bill Edmonds, their NSW branch Corporate Relations and Communications Manager:

Tim: Why can't I call myself a diabetic?

Bill: Well you can, obviously. I can't remember exactly when it was changed, but there's been a move around the world over the last ten years towards being politically correct—that you don't want to be an 'ic' any more, a 'diabetic'. We don't call someone with cancer a 'canceric', and you're not a 'leukemic', or a 'lymphonic'. So it was felt, why label someone with diabetes and turn the person who has the disease into the disease? So most of the carers, doctors, diabetes educators, dietitians and the people who are involved in the team, are changing from using 'diabetic' to 'A person who has diabetes'. Diabetic is still being used, but I would say, in a few years' time, it is likely to be used less and less.

Tim: But somebody would say, 'I'm an alcoholic', with pride at an Alcoholics Anonymous meeting. Like diabetes it's something that is always there. Once an alcoholic, always an alcoholic.

Bill: Well I think that's changing too. I heard an interview the other day with a doctor who said, 'You're not actually an alcoholic, you're a person with an alcohol problem . . . '

Tim: It's the same thing.

Bill: Yes, but I think there is a general trend—it's all in the political correctness. Until someone actually mentions it, you don't bother to think about that. People these days don't say you're deaf, they say you've got a hearing problem. They don't say you're blind, you've got a sight problem.

Tim: Well I'm deaf as well as diabetic! However, on reflection, I'm not fat—only circumferentially challenged.

Bill: Naturally . . .

Dr Norman Swan, presenter of ABC Radio National *Health Report*, strongly suggested that I interview Professor Lesley Campbell, who as well as being Professor of Medicine at the University of New South Wales, is the Director of the Diabetes Centre at St Vincent's Hospital in Sydney, and Principal Research Fellow at the Garvan Institute of Medical Research. (I didn't dare ask what she did in her spare time.) Lesley Campbell has published a truly astonishing number of research papers on diabetes, and I wanted to ask her about the latest medical developments in the treatment of diabetes and would there ever be a cure—and if so how far off that might be?

But naturally I started off talking about myself:

Tim: Lesley, I know everyone says this, but why me? I didn't think I was living all that indulgently. I exercised, was a bit overweight. I'm 66 years old with absolutely no history of diabetes on either side of my family.

Lesley: Why did fate do this to you? I think sometimes it's hard for us to know our family history as accurately as we might want to. I still say the most common reason for people to have diabetes is that they have what we call polygenes—they have an assortment of genes that predispose them to diabetes. Sometimes there have been early deaths in the family of the people who gave them some of that assortment of genes. So it's not a single gene that can be traced relatively easily, for example like childhood fibrocystic disease. Diabetes appears late and there are many genes involved which we haven't identified. So often you'll have an Aunty Flo who could have been run over by a car before she actually got diabetes—therefore you don't know that she could have got diabetes.

Tim: So there has to be a genetic component?

Lesley: Not absolutely, but the theory is that you have a predisposition in your genes—at least that's the one I hold to. There are other causes, alcohol being one. I don't want to cast nasty aspersions here.

Tim: I *am* a journalist!

Lesley: That's true, actually. I have known some journalists in my time, you've raised an interesting point there. But I'm becoming more and more convinced that even when there's an obvious precipitant some people are more predisposed by underlying genetics. I may be a little biased to this view, but there'd be very few people who would completely discount genetics, in the sense that there's a predisposition first, then your environment comes along and determines when you get diabetes, what age you get it and perhaps how severely you get it.

Tim: So, if I had been a better Vegemite, not drunk so much and perhaps been more careful about what I ate, might I have put off getting Type 2?

Lesley: Exactly. You might have waited until you were 92!

Tim: But I'd have got Type 2 eventually?

Lesley: At 92 because, let me put it this way, there are a lot of genes for diabetes around. That's another interesting thing. Why are there so many genes for it? These are not necessarily 'bad' genes—they're the survival genes. Some of the genes that predispose you to having diabetes are the ones that cause people to have fat around their middles and conserve fat. Man's whole history has been concerned with starvation and war. To survive those extreme circumstances, the genes that predispose people to conserve energy and to keep it in an energy store that is easy to mobilise—those genes are 'good' genes. The abdominal fat store is exactly that sort of fat store—so you can put it down easily and you can mobilise it fast for exercising the muscles to run away from wild animals or to gather food. However, if you're just lying around watching television, it turns into a nasty fat store because it tends to lead to a thing called insulin resistance and can predispose people both to being fatter and also to probably having diabetes, it may even clog up their pancreas. That's a theory, but it's a working theory.

Tim: I hear it's happening to quite young children now—pre-pubescents and adolescents?

Lesley: Exactly. It's underactivity, because we were meant to chase our food, run it to the ground and then eat it. Now it's being delivered to the door by the delivery man. So we've got two things—easy access to the food and lack of physical activity in getting the food. So we've got the genes for storing it and mobilising it rapidly, then what's happened is we've been tricked by our working masters who want us to sit in front of a computer instead.

Tim: Well that's certainly what I did. Are any forms of exercise better than others?

Lesley: I think it's important to choose an exercise that has a purpose. If we have good survival genes, why would you waste yourself just running up and down on the spot doing nothing? I think we are meant to be doing exercise that gets you somewhere. I always advise people to do exercise that is meaningful. It's better if they can walk to and from work, or do some shopping. If they can incorporate exercise in their lifestyle it's more likely to be something that will be a permanent change rather just exercise for the sake of doing it.

Tim: I suppose I do that with my 45-minute walk along the back of the beach every morning to get the paper.

Lesley: Well that's part of your life. If getting your paper is part of your 'killing of your animal' and that's all you've got, that's fine. At least you can see a purpose to what you are doing. I rather worry that the gym—which is what has become the replacement—often seems futile. Sometimes people don't even walk to it, they drive. Some people will wait for the bus to pick them up to take them to their gymnastics, so they don't go there any more after a while.

Tim: What is so good about exercise for people with diabetes?

Lesley: Because it burns sugar without using insulin. It also burns off fat, so in a way it makes the body more sensitive to insulin. Those metabolic things help to reverse the abnormalities that diabetes has burdened you with. And it helps in weight loss. For people who want not only to lose weight but to keep it off, ongoing activity helps to do this.

Tim: Several people I've spoken to—Eva Cox for one—is cross about the tendency for people to be censorious about diabetes. 'You brought this on yourself because of your lifestyle.' There seems to be a culture of blame.

Lesley: Well I think this is one of the terrible things for people with Type 2, the misery that can hit you when you consider all the awful things that can happen to you because of complications—affecting your cardiovascular system, your eyesight, and the list goes on. Then you walk around and people look at you and say, 'It's your fault you've got this disease'. But there really isn't evidence for that. The evidence is that you actually carry some fantastically good genes and when Mr Bush and Mr Howard have really got things going badly economically, you'll be the ones that will make it because you've actually got these genes for survival—that is for fat storing. They are the same genes that keep people from losing weight in times of famine.

Tim: But then again weight is not good?

Lesley: It depends under what circumstances. Excess weight is not good in general, but the genes that cause it would be good in extreme hard times. But in 'normal' urban living, they also cause diabetes to be so prevalent. It isn't gorging, it isn't gluttony. People don't want diabetes, they don't want the weight. It's absurd to blame diabetic people.

So now I don't have to blame myself, just Aunt Flo (it would help if I had an aunt so called). However, I do find it curious, that in this day and age with so many medical breakthroughs on so many fronts, that diabetes is still regarded as incurable.

I asked Professor Lesley Campbell why a 'cure' was so elusive, and what hope lay ahead for people with Type 2 diabetes on the medical front?

Lesley: I have great hope. There are very good treatments available already—particularly to control blood sugar. There is a bit of a problem that some of the treatments cause weight gain—but not all of them. Going on to insulin causes most Type 2s to gain weight, and that is well known. Some of the newer drugs are quite promising, and may even help prevent people moving from the stage of pre-diabetes—insulin resistance—to developing Type 2.

Then of course there are treatments. Eye disease is now under better control; so is kidney disease and blood pressure. Not so long ago people used to die of high blood pressure, It used to be hard to get them under control quickly when I first graduated. I remember one case at Sydney Hospital, when a man with extremely high blood pressure went home to get his things, came back and had a stroke before we could get his blood pressure controlled. Now we have four or five types of drugs that are excellent for reducing blood pressure, and as a side benefit, also reduce strokes and heart attacks. We're not doing enough yet, but it just seems the better the blood pressure, the less heart disease. So with really good control and good outcomes we'll all certainly be living longer. In fact you'll have to be beaten to death with a stick eventually because there's just so much evidence for better outcomes from all these different treatments compounding in different studies.

Tim: But will there be a 'cure' for Type 2 diabetes?

Lesley: I think insight into what's causing Type 2 must be at least ten years away.

Tim: Is that going to involve mucking around with genes or what?

Lesley: I don't think we'll actually do it by genes. I think we'll get drugs and treatments from knowing what the genes are. When you think about how the public is behaving about genetically modifying a piece of canola . . . but we'll get good drugs out of it.

Tim: So you're optimistic about that?

Lesley: I'm optimistic about great insights into good drug prevention—as we have for a lot of other diseases that we had to treat with diet. Take cholesterol for instance. Perhaps partly as a result of our lifestyles, everyone was trying diets to get their cholesterol levels down. Now there's a drug that you just swallow and nobody talks about cholesterol a great deal these days.

Tim: What is the future do you think for people with Type 1 diabetes?

Lesley: Medical researchers have always promised poor Type 1s that a solution was just around the corner. I get very upset about that because there's nothing more desperate than the parents of a Type 1. I've watched that for 25 years, people promising Type 1s, particularly parents of Type 1s, that there is a breakthrough for their young children. However, the possibility of successful transplants is becoming closer now. One type of transplant in particular is finally looking like it might be more successful because the drugs to prevent rejection are less toxic.

Tim: Are you speaking of pancreas transplants?

Lesley: Yes. They infuse the cells down the portal vein. Again you've got to take them from cadaveric transplants but it's a breakthrough that hasn't been successful before. There are now trials going on across the world. The transplant of a whole pancreas has been successful in people who also need a kidney transplant. I was among a team that worked on an artificial pancreas when I first came to St Vincent's 24 years ago, and I personally know machinery will not replace the brilliant pancreas because the algorithms and the fail-safe things that the pancreas do are just too hard. They're still trying to do that, though.

I think the future for Type 1s is transplantation and, again, drugs. I think breaking the immune codes and so on will probably get closer in ten or twenty years. So I'd say if you wanted to forecast the next big thing—it would most likely be transplantation.

With no immediate quick fixes on the medical drawing boards, prevention is the only alternative to a cure—although that, sadly, cannot be so for those with Type 1. For those who are teetering on the brink of Type 2 diabetes, in that pre-diabetes phase when it is possible to pull back from the full-blown disease, there *are* options. These involve all those obvious but difficult to achieve things such as a healthy lifestyle, losing weight, eating the right food, exercising and not thrashing the grog as though there were no tomorrows.

These are public health issues, and they are difficult to sell not only to the punters, but to governments, for whom you'd think the prospect of cutting back on those horrendous health budgets would be attractive. But as a society we are heavily hooked on going to our doctors when we get sick and expecting a pill to be prescribed to put us right. This is enthusiastically supported by the drug companies, who spend huge amounts promoting their products, to doctors as well as to consumers through general advertising. The Federal Government assists this process by allocating and subsidising certain selected drugs on to the Pharmaceutical Benefits Scheme, which makes them available to the general public at an affordable price. The drug companies compete keenly for these subsidised cash cows to boost their profits. This well entrenched cycle makes it exceedingly difficult to attract Federal Government funding for public health campaigns. The hospital system and general practitioners are barely managing to cope with a flood of patients presenting with easily preventable conditions. Dare I mention smoking for one?

Diabetes and diabetes related conditions are a big ticket budget item. The cost of Type 2 alone is estimated at three billion dollars a year. With 1.2 million Australians with diabetes—and half of them unaware of their condition—early detection could stave off some very expensive complications. So you'd think that in 2003 when Diabetes Australia–NSW came up with a proposal for a campaign, tied to Diabetes Week, to find that hidden half-a-million-odd Australians who had diabetes but didn't know it, that both the Federal and State governments might have thought it a worthwhile investment. Absolutely not! Neither the Federal or NSW State governments were interested at the time. The reason given, if it wasn't so serious, would be a subject for satire. The Federal government balked because it didn't want a national, mass-appeal awareness campaign! It has since, however, provided funding for a state-based campaign.

At the time, Diabetes Australia–NSW CEO, Liz Peers,

expressed disappointment in the decision and spelt out the official response:

> The Government was concerned our campaign would put a strain on the public health system, which is struggling to cope with the number of existing diabetes cases.

Dare one ask about the consequences in future years? That was never addressed.

Diabetes Australia–NSW went ahead and did what they could themselves to spread the message about the fastest growing chronic disease in the world today. Nevertheless, it is a hard message to sell, as Bill Edmonds, Corporate Relations and Communications Manager of Diabetes Australia–NSW, makes clear: 'How do you get people to think about a disease that they can't feel, when there are no signs of illness and they don't feel crook?' Over the past two to three years there has been a change in tactics to get the message about diabetes problems through:

Bill: Years ago they used to show pictures of missing feet, and people with diabetes who had eyesight and other problems and really concentrated on shock tactics. But it didn't work. The diabetes numbers showed no sign of going down. There was no recognition of the problem. I used to say to friends of mine in the diabetes community, 'You've got to come up with another way to get people to think about diabetes'. They said, 'If you're so smart, you do it'. So I spent a lot of time thinking of how to get people to think about diabetes. I did surveys and people would say, 'I don't want to know if I've got diabetes, don't tell me. I'm healthy, I'm not feeling crook'. How do you get them to think about the day when they will be sick?

Tim: Which is an almost impossible task isn't it?

Bill: Many of my colleagues thought so! But we did come up with a radical new approach. The essence of it was, don't try and get people to think about disease, or about the possibility of being ill, get them to think about being *well.* If you look around there are indicators of your health, you use them all the time, like your cholesterol levels or your iron levels. If you've got a headache you take a tablet because there's an indicator that things aren't going so well. So I looked at it and thought, 'The only way you're going to discover whether you have diabetes is to have a blood test'. If you've got high cholesterol, or high blood pressure, we know that most people do something about it. This happened to me.

My doctor discovered I had high cholesterol, and recommended I do something about it, so I started an exercise program. About six months later I went for another test and he said, 'You've reduced your risk level from 150 per cent to 10 per cent so you're on the chart to doing better'. I adopted that same principle into the diabetes area and said, 'People should know their blood glucose level'.

We did a lot of research and we found that people, once they were told that there was this thing called blood glucose—they hadn't heard of it before—said, 'We want to know about it'. So in 2001 we launched the 'Be well, know your BGL' campaign, telling people to find out about their BGL the next time they visited their doctor. That's changed a lot of perceptions, because many people are now saying, 'Yes, I should know my blood glucose level'.

Tim: But the slogan, 'Be well, know your BGL', wouldn't mean anything to people would it?

Bill: Exactly—that's just the point. It was designed to stimulate their interest. To change their behaviour. When we launched the 'Be well, know your BGL' campaign we got phone calls from a few people saying that we didn't tell them what BGL was. I said that it was deliberately designed to do that. 'Now you're ringing up and asking about BGL. You'd never heard of it before. Now please discuss it with your doctor.'

Three years ago, before that campaign started, we did a survey and only between 25 and 33 per cent of people said they had heard of this thing called 'blood glucose level'. Yet those same people knew about blood cholesterol and were aware their blood pressure was important—some 70 to 80 per cent knew that. They knew two indicators of their health but they didn't know the third. We did a survey just before our more recent pre-diabetes campaign and it shows you how it's changed. Now 80 per cent of the people we sampled knew about blood glucose and that they should find out about it. So within a two-year period, we'd got people thinking about knowing their blood glucose level, without knowing whether they had diabetes. That is how we began to turn that lack of awareness around.

Unawareness of diabetes is dangerous for everyone

As a new chum I am more aware than most about how much I didn't know about diabetes, and my interest is now certainly more than academic. This issue goes beyond the statistic of half the people in Australia with diabetes not knowing that they have it. Even with the best will in the world, those with Type 1 diabetes, and those with Type 2 who are either on medication or insulin, may miscalculate their carbohydrate and insulin balance, and become distressed and ill in a public place. They may lose consciousness altogether.

My New Zealand friend, Bob—previously mentioned in chapter one—recently had an unpleasant episode with high blood sugar. He journeyed from the Land of the Short Flat Vowel to Australia to attend the funeral of a friend and former journalist colleague but came perilously close to needing a funeral organised for him. Travel in itself can cause established routines to go awry. Bob, an insulin-dependent Type 2, managed to leave En Zed without packing his blood testing meter. He guessed his insulin requirements and got it wrong. 'I had absolutely no memory', he told me later, 'of the day of the funeral and most of the next. I collapsed and became part of a kind of "pass the parcel" game until I got back to my hotel and eventually on the plane back to New Zealand'. He was met by a medical team, who stabilised him, and sent him home in a wheelchair. It had been a near run thing. Bob admitted that it wasn't terribly smart to fly overseas without his glucometer.

At least Bob was among friends who were aware he had diabetes. The experience of Cherie Evans, a mother of two who had a hypo in a supermarket in Wellington, New South Wales, is the stuff nightmares are made of—but it was sadly real. The story was reported in the Diabetes Australia–NSW publication, *Issues*, Autumn 2002.

Cherie Evans has had Type 1 diabetes for 17 years. Although she tested her blood sugar before beginning her supermarket shopping—it was 8.5 mmol/L—she became confused, light-headed, hot and shaky while pushing a heavy trolley up and down the aisles. Feeling unwell, she sat down in the aisle and tested her blood sugar—a worryingly low 2.9 mmol/L. Her symptoms became even worse at the checkout, and she mentioned to the cashier that she thought she was having a hypo.

She paid for her shopping and went to her car, where she sat eating some lollies to try and get her BGL back to normal levels. Two shop security guards approached her, accused her of not paying for her shopping and demanded she accompany them back to the store where she was questioned and her bags searched. She knew her blood glucose level was dangerously low, and she begged the security guards to get her some honey. But Ms Evans claimed they ignored her request, assuming her slurred speech, confusion, shakiness and slow mannerisms were because she was drunk. 'They told me a strong cup of coffee, "Would sober me up".'

Cherie Evans explained she had insulin-dependent diabetes and was having a hypo. 'I pleaded with them to call my doctor who was just up the road.' Instead they called the police, who arrested her. (A couple of small items had fallen under her bags in the trolley at the checkout—worth only a few dollars. Ms Evans explained that she had been unwell and hadn't noticed what happened at the checkout.) At Wellington Police Station she was locked in a cell without her handbag containing her glucose sweets, insulin and blood glucose meter. No medical help was offered, as Cherie Evans said later in court, because the police assumed she was drunk. The police later defended their actions, saying it was normal practice to remove personal effects from all prisoners while in custody, even those with diabetes.

The case came to Wellington local court in November 2002, and was quickly thrown out. The blood glucose meter record, stored in its memory, was definitive evidence of Cherie Evans's hypo. But seven months later Ms Evans was still having counselling and medication for depression and panic attacks. 'I was so humiliated', she said. 'Now I am so terrified of having a hypo I won't go out alone.'

Diabetes Australia–NSW took up her case with the New South Wales Police and the Anti-Discrimination Board. It is a sorry tale, but not an unusual one, alas, because of the low public awareness of diabetes in our community. Perhaps it is fear of discrimination, or it may be other factors which make many people who have diabetes unwilling to make their condition known outside their immediate family—perhaps not even to friends. It is something I raised with Bill Edmonds, Corporate Relations and Communications Manager of Diabetes Australia–NSW:

Tim: How would you describe the status of somebody with diabetes, Bill? Is it something that's brushed under the carpet or are people prepared to say, without much fuss, 'Yeah, I've got diabetes'?

Bill: In many cases people with diabetes don't like to admit it. There is a stigma attached, and it's a pity that there are not more people in the public arena that openly talk about it, whether it's Type 1 or Type 2. We know high corporate-level people who are Type 1, who won't admit to their bosses and to the organisation that they've got Type 1 diabetes because they think that it impairs their chances of being promoted through the business. They fear that bosses will think they will become a burden, that they won't be able to travel because of restrictions covering people with Type 1.

Tim: And for those with Type 2?

Bill: Type 2s generally keep quiet about their condition too. We know a lot of high-profile people with Type 2 diabetes and there's a stigma attached to that. We don't yet have an open enough society willing to talk about it, although I think it's changing. In the last couple of years there has been an increase in the obesity debate, and the understanding that it's a lifestyle problem, not a stigma attached problem, and there are family histories to it. So I think it's slowly changing, but not as quickly as we'd like. In England, as you probably know, they have high-profile entertainers and celebrities—like the late Sir Harry Secombe—who represent the diabetes organisations over there and talk frankly and honestly about diabetes. We haven't yet reached that open stage here but I think it is changing. The crazy part about it is, 80 to 90 per cent of the people diagnosed with diabetes, or who are obese or overweight, are walking around, in most cases, as a visual display that they've probably got a diabetes problem, if not now but later.

People don't like to admit, 'Yes I contributed to my own diabetes condition by not looking after myself, by letting myself get overweight or fat, and leading the good life'. I think it is changing, but certainly not as quickly as we would like. We have approached a number of prominent people who we know have diabetes and asked them to talk about it, but they won't. It is helpful to us when they do, and some people—may I say like you—do help us to get our message out into the community.

Tim: What about actual discrimination towards people with diabetes?

Bill: Well I think one of the reasons people don't want to talk openly about it, is because of the discrimination. Insurance is a huge problem. If you've got diabetes and you want life insurance, then most insurance companies—just about every insurance company that we know of—will either make the premiums prohibitively high or they won't insure you at all. Now it doesn't matter to them whether you've got well-managed diabetes, or whether your diabetes is out of control.

Tim: Type 1, Type 2?

Bill: It doesn't matter, because they lump it all in together—they only consider the actuarial figures and look at everyone across the board, they don't look at individual cases. Now we think we have organised a breakthrough after two years of negotiations with a broker. We've just made an arrangement where we've got an insurance company that will look at each person's individual case, and give them insurance cover based on that.

Tim: What typically happens to someone who develops Type 2 diabetes in later life and tries to get insurance?

Bill: The biggest problem we've got—and we see it quite often—is with the person who's, say, getting to 50 or 55 and just lost their job or is changing jobs and decides they want to start up the business they've always wanted, to run the bookstore down the road or the little travel agency. He or she gets their superannuation, or payout. It's not enough to buy the business, so they go to the bank to borrow more money and the bank says, 'Sure, we'll lend you the money. All you need is a health check'. The health check discovers that the applicant has got diabetes and that's the end of the insurance and the loan. We have heard of these cases, time and time again.

Insurance is probably the number one complaint. Of course there are complaints from people who work in various high-profile jobs, police and the defence forces—we're getting situations now where cooks and clerks who are nowhere near a battle front are being dismissed from the defence force because they have diabetes and *might* be involved in crucial battlefield decisions. That's one argument currently going on with the Defence Department.

Tim: Is this Type 2 you're talking about?

Bill: Type 2 or Type 1, it doesn't matter, it's basically diabetes. In one case we had a discussion with a large library in Sydney where a Type 1 person was spending many hours doing research in the library and wasn't allowed to take any food in. We had to ring up the library and say, 'We know this person. Is it okay to take in an orange juice and a sandwich so she can eat to help manage her diabetes?' We have problems with children. We had a letter the other day from a little kid, saying she was diagnosed with Type 1 and some of the kids at school were teasing and bullying her, calling her a diseased person. So you come back to this phrase about whether you're a 'diabetic' or 'a person with diabetes'. It starts at an early age as demonstrated by this little girl who was so distraught about the discrimination against her because she had diabetes. I mean, kids are so cruel, pointing the finger and saying, 'You're a diseased person'. But then again many adults in the general community aren't all that good about understanding diabetes either. There's still a long way to go.

The long road ahead

It is now a year since I was diagnosed with Type 2 diabetes. Having uttered the usual despairing wail, 'Why me?', I now know that my diabetes is not entirely my fault—the yet-to-be identified Aunt Flo can carry her fair genetic share of the blame. But there is also no doubt that I almost certainly arrived some years earlier at the diabetes' gates than I needed to by the unrestrained way I stuffed food down my throat, lashed into the demon drink and exercised intermittently.

After being confirmed with Type 2, I went through all the classic stages of grief, anger, self-pity (Ros soon snapped me out of that) and the gloomy prognostication that life was going to be pretty damn dull on a diet without rich cheeses, puddings and second helpings. I soon realised there were lots of tasty, good things to eat, and some of the forbidden goodies could still be had as an occasional tasty treat. Sweet things were okay in moderation and I did not have to be a diet martyr. I drink two to three glasses of wine in the evening (I'm still dinkering with the idea of those alcohol-free days) and occasionally a bit more if the occasion demands.

At ten kilos lighter I feel better than I have in years, and my blood glucose is mostly in the normal range, between 4 to 8 mmol/L. My fasting readings in the morning are slightly higher than normal—straying from the 5 into the 6 mmol/L range. But that isn't surprising, seeing as I do have Type 2 diabetes. The results from the all important three-monthly HbA1c test are well and truly in the 'normal' range. In fact I have brought it down a few percentage points. At one stage I had it as low as 5.1 per cent. Anything over 7 would be a cause of concern.

I'm on tablets to keep my cholesterol and blood pressure down, but so far I do not need any medication for my diabetes. My GP, Ron, seems confident I will have several more years in this happy state of affairs. But I know that eventually my poor overworked pancreas will tire of pumping out insulin that is being poorly processed by my body, and it will need some assistance. And if I stray from the true path of sensible diet and physical activity I will progress to medication much more quickly.

Having talked to many of my friends and acquaintances who have diabetes in various degrees of severity, I realise I am one of the lucky ones. I've always been a fairly positive person anyway, and I feel optimistic about my future, such as it is at the fairly ripe age of 66. It may well be that being diagnosed with Type 2 was a wake-up call for me to take better care of my one-only-issue body.

Diabetes is not one of those conditions that can be treated by drugs—or insulin—alone. Each individual can exert an enormous influence on their own health and well-being through sensible eating and exercise. As Dr Ron reminded me, people with diabetes who manage to pull their HbA1c rating back by even .7 of a per cent get quite remarkable benefits to their health.

I suppose the main message that has come through to me during my first year with Type 2 diabetes is the concept of 'control'. That is all you can do with diabetes, you can't beat it. But *you* can take control of it, and no doctor or dietitian or diabetic educator can do that for you. They can help, with advice and prescriptions for drugs, but they can only work within the limits of your own self-control and will to give your body the best fighting chance against this malevolent enemy. So much depends on what people with diabetes do for themselves.

I think it helps to talk things over with other Type 2s from time to time, and to attend the occasional refresher lecture at a diabetes health centre. It is also essential—in my view—to keep testing your BGL twice daily, even if you are turning in close to normal readings. Not only does it help you monitor your own situation (so you can perhaps pull back after some indulgent gastronomic excesses), it also gives your doctor a continuing series of snapshots on how you are fairing so he can quickly spot any changes.

It hasn't happened to me yet, but I understand that if you are ill with the 'flu—for example—or just stressed, your blood glucose rises. And if it rises for no apparent reason and stays high, your doctor will want to know. If you don't test regularly, you won't be able to alert your medical advisers. Sure, you'll have to miss some testing days because of travel or a hectic schedule, but be conscious of that and make sure you do it the following day. It doesn't pay to get too cocky, though I was having a good run of BGL figures recently and went out to a friend's sixtieth birthday. (At my age you alternate between significant decade-marking birthdays and funerals.) I tucked into everything as if there was no tomorrow, just like the bad old days. The alcohol, perversely, kept my BGL reading late that night at a moderate 6.4 mmol/L. My fasting reading the next morning was in the high sixes (not good). That evening, two hours after a distinctly more diabetes friendly evening meal, I was 7.8 mmol/L—which is getting close to the naughty range. I immediately became a good person, exercised and ate sensibly and soon had myself back down to random tests of fives and sixes again. It was a reminder that a run of 'normal' BGL figures doesn't mean that diabetes has magically gone away.

One year on, in some trepidation, I fronted up to my GP for my fourth ever HbA1c test—the one that catches you out if you have been fudging your blood glucose level figures! As previously mentioned, your blood cells live for 90 days which provides a built-in record of your BGLs. This test rates you on a scale between 1 and 10. Anything over 7 is a worry and would indicate the end of my 'diet and exercise' period, and would probably mean some kind of medication. My first HbA1c test came in at 5.6 per cent, which wasn't too bad really, and within the 'normal' range. The lower you can get your rating, the less chance of side effects and complications. I pegged it back to 5.5, and even down as low as 5.1, so I felt a bit smug. But that's a dangerous emotion when dealing with the unpredictability of diabetes. The last HbA1c test, just before this book went to press, was 5.4 which meant I was losing ground, but still well within the comfort zone. I also noticed that my fasting morning readings had crept up from the mid to high 5 mmol/L range, into the 6s over the previous four months, occasionally straying into the low 7s. Normal people would have fasting readings in the low to mid 5s. This is a sign, of course, that I do have Type 2 diabetes. My GP, Ron, says that some people have cyclic rises and falls in their HbA1c tests at different times of the year. Only time will tell whether I am heading towards having to take medication for my diabetes sooner rather than later.

I don't think about my diabetes all the time now. But I do when I prick the side of my finger for the daily blood tests, and that is good. We need to be aware. Type 2 diabetes does not interfere unduly with my life—at least for the time being I control it, it doesn't control me. I've met some people—Geoff, for instance, in chapter four—who, through no fault of their own, are having tough and stressful times with see-sawing blood glucose levels and associated complications. I often think there is little justice when it comes to matters of health, and I don't mean just diabetes. But a positive attitude is known to be beneficial when tackling any illness, and that is certainly true for Geoff who faces each day with great courage and optimism. Positive thinking may even lower your blood glucose!

One year on I can honestly say I've stopped saying, 'This can't happen to me!' The way things have turned out I feel I have every reason to say, 'Lucky me'.

Suggested reading

Diabetes & You—The Essential Guide, Diabetes Australia.

Diabetes at Your Fingertips—All Your Questions Answered about Living With Diabetes, Professor Peter Sönksen, Dr Charles Fox, Sue Judd with Diabetes Australia, McGraw Hill, 1998.

Diabetes for Dummies, Alan L. Rubin (adapted by Professor Lesley Campbell and the Diabetes Centre St Vincent's Hospital, Sydney), Hungry Minds, 2003.

The New Glucose Revolution—The Glycemic Index Solution for Maximum Health, Jennie Brand-Miller, Kaye Foster-Powell, Assoc. Prof. Stephen Colagiuri, Hodder Headline Australia, 2003.

Preamble: The History of Diabetes, D. A. Pyke, John Wiley & Sons Ltd, 1999.

Sweet & Sour—A Diabetic Life, Peter Corris, Southern Cross University Press, 2000.

Understanding Diabetes—Managing Your Life with Diabetes, The Diabetes Centre St Vincent's Hospital, Sydney, Simon & Schuster, 1997.

Printed in Dunstable, United Kingdom

88190715R00129